The Oxygen Legacy

A Fountain of Youth and An End to All Disease

With Best wishes to Janice and Nick Triantos for a longer, healthier and happier life —
Tom Tasseff
(Oct. 7, 2012)

Thomas Tasseff

outskirtspress
DENVER, COLORADO

The opinions expressed in this manuscript are solely the opinions of the author and do not represent the opinions or thoughts of the publisher. The author has represented and warranted full ownership and/or legal right to publish all the materials in this book.

The Oxygen Legacy:
A Fountain of Youth and An End to All Disease
All Rights Reserved.
Copyright © 2012 Thomas Tasseff
v1.0

Cover Photo © 2012 Alexandra (Tasseff) Brunelle. All rights reserved - used with permission.

This book may not be reproduced, transmitted, or stored in whole or in part by any means, including graphic, electronic, or mechanical without the express written consent of the publisher except in the case of brief quotations embodied in critical articles and reviews.

Outskirts Press, Inc.
http://www.outskirtspress.com

ISBN: 978-1-4327-9564-1

Library of Congress Control Number: 2012911259

Outskirts Press and the "OP" logo are trademarks belonging to Outskirts Press, Inc.

PRINTED IN THE UNITED STATES OF AMERICA

*I wish to express my sincere gratitude
and dedicate this book to my dear wife, Nada,
to my three children, Clint, Maria, and Alexandra,
and to my seven grandchildren,
Athan, Athena, Paul, Holly, Andrew,
Nicholas, and Alexis.*

*I further dedicate this book to
the 175 million Americans who will
so needlessly die of cancer and other horrible
but entirely preventable diseases in the near future*

*Finally, I dedicate this book to the 300 million living
Americans who will sadly lose so many loved ones in
the next few years, but who can do something to prevent
these horrible deaths by living longer, healthier, and
happier lives...
beginning right now!*

*It is You to whom I dedicate this book...
My Continuing Legacy to You!*

Contents

Foreword: The Oxygen Legacy Begins i
Introduction: A Legacy of Good Health Continues v
Preface.. ix
Acknowledgements.. xiii
Chapter 1   Our Body is a Precision
                Electronic Machine 1
Chapter 2   Antioxidants and Free Radicals............... 13
Chapter 3   Astaxanthin: The Alpha Antioxidant...... 27
Chapter 4   Our Links to Aging................................ 31
Chapter 5   Discovery of an All-Natural
                Anti-Aging Formula............................... 49
Chapter 6   Our Body and DNA................................ 53
Chapter 7   The Cause of Cancer
                and Every Other Disease 67
Chapter 8   DCA: A "Magic Bullet" Cure for Cancer.. 81
Chapter 9   Lyme Disease:
                Difficult to Detect and Treat 105

Chapter 10	Memory Loss and Mental Decline	111
Chapter 11	Alzheimer's and Organic Virgin Cocoanut Oil	123
Chapter 12	Celiac Disease and Gluten Sensitivity	133
Chapter 13	Latent Cancer	143
Chapter 14	The FDA and Its Approved Cancer Drug: Avastin	149
Conclusion	A Legacy of Oxygen for You	155
Postscript: Disclaimer, Recommendations, and		159
About The Author		163
Bibliography: References Cited and Sources of Further Information		167
Books by Tom Tasseff:		173

Foreword:
The Oxygen Legacy Begins

Four and a half billion years ago, the Sun, the Moon, the Earth, and all of the other planets in our Solar System coalesced from an accumulation of physical debris produced during the giant cosmic explosion of matter and energy now universally known as the Big Bang.

Oxygen in its elemental form (O) was, of course, present in many of the rocks, minerals, and gasses generated by that cataclysmic genesis and subsequent planetary accretion; but it was not the molecular form of oxygen (O_2) that we now know of and upon which we have since come to depend.

Sometime between one and a half and three billion years ago, life arose from the primordial molecular soup by the processes of organic evolution and perhaps with help from the introduction of large biomolecules. Many scientists now believe that some large biomolecules came to Earth from previously existing organisms and organic molecules reigned in from the cosmos as evidenced by their presence in asteroids and in meteorites from space.

These early forms of life still did not use oxygen; and molecular oxygen (O_2) was actually toxic (oxidizing) to their existence for another billion years. Then, about two and a half billion years ago, one group of these simple single-celled organisms evolved an amazing new process for converting and metabolizing energy from their environment and for creating their own food... Photosynthesis.

Photosynthesis is the process whereby many living things, especially green plants, take in water and carbon dioxide (CO_2) in the presence of sunlight and chlorophyll to synthesize simple sugars, which they then use as a source of energy for all of their metabolic processes. These early photosynthesizers gave off molecular oxygen (O_2) as a metabolic waste product and oxygen remained toxic to life for another billion years.

Elemental iron (Fe) was abundantly dissolved in the seawater of the early Earth. As the newly formed molecular oxygen (O_2) bubbled up through the water column, it combined with the dissolved iron and formed the red-orange oxide of iron that we call rust. As iron oxide (FeO_2) formed, it precipitated out of the seawater and accumulated at the bottom of the seas in thick sedimentary deposits, which we now actively and economically mine as iron ore.

By about two billion years ago, photosynthesis had produced sufficient molecular oxygen to "rust" all of the dissolved iron out of the seas. The evidence of this is that all iron ore deposits are about two billion years old and none is any younger.

With all of the iron atoms thus otherwise occupied, oxygen was then free to accumulate in the atmosphere. Since oxygen was still toxic, living things had to either adapt to it or die. Because life is exceedingly resilient, it quickly evolved a means to use oxygen actively as a final acidic hydrogen ion ($H+$) acceptor in many of life's metabolic processes. Oxygen has since become crucial to respiration, the process of efficiently converting food to energy in most living things. We now cannot live without oxygen, and generally speaking, the more the better.

In this book, Tom Tasseff shares with you what he has learned from a lifetime of research and experience on the benefits of optimizing oxygen intake and sustaining efficient nutritionally based aerobic (oxygen) metabolism as both a potential Fountain of Youth and an End to ALL Disease. This book, ***The Oxygen Legacy***, is Tom Tasseff's continuing legacy of good health, long life, and happiness to you.

Steven J. Wamback, Editor

Introduction:
A Legacy of Good Health Continues

The Oxygen Legacy:
A Fountain of Youth and an End to All Disease
(Thomas Tasseff, 2012, Outskirts Press, Inc.)

In this, my third book and continuing legacy to you, I wish to share with you, my readers what I believe to be some of the most important lifesaving strategies that I have learned through research and personal experience in my 81 (and still counting!) years of life. I introduced some of these concepts to you in my first two books,

Win The Ultimate Battle For Your Health:
The Lifesaving Legacy of Tom Tasseff
(Thomas Tasseff, 2008, Outskirts Press, Inc.)

Live Forever (Or at Least to 100):
More Lifesaving Strategies from Tom Tasseff
(Thomas Tasseff, 2010, Outskirts Press, Inc.)

Throughout this trilogy of good health, long life, and happiness, my continuing legacy to you, I have attempted to share with you some of the key concepts that you can actively employ to improve the quality and length of your life through good health practices, better nutrition, and taking personal responsibility for your health, your happiness, and your life.

Some of these concepts and practices that I have introduced might be considered as "health secrets". Secrets… not because they cannot be known… but because mainstream medicine and big pharmaceutical corporations actively try to prevent you from knowing these things; and because in the overall scheme of things and particularly in our greed-based economy, disease and especially cancer… Pays!

As you read this book and take personal responsibility for your health, I hope you will carefully scrutinize the objectives of big medicine and big pharmaceuticals by doing your homework, conducting your own research, and taking the word of the "powers that be" with no more than a grain of salt.

I urge you to proceed with the knowledge that monetary

profits and financial gain are often their primary motives… not your good health or your best interests. ***YOU*** and you alone have the power and the responsibility to take charge of your health, your life, and your destiny.

Tom Tasseff, 2012

Preface

My intention in writing this book is to share with you what I have learned and employed in winning the ultimate battle for my own health as based upon a lifetime of good living, from conducting my own in-depth research, and from the experience of overcoming my own health obstacles. My continuing legacy to you is to provide you with the ammunition that I have found available and have used to improve my own general health and happiness.

It is my hope that as you read this book, you will do so with an open mind and find both the information and the inspiration to continue to do your own research, to seek appropriate and cooperative professional medical health care consultation as necessary, and to make informed decisions that will lead you to a healthier and happier life.

None of the information provided nor any of the opinions

expressed in this publication should be construed as personal medical advice or instruction. No action should be taken based solely upon on the contents of this book. Readers are advised to consult their own appropriate health care professionals on any matters relating to their personal medical health, health concerns, symptoms, illness, disease, or treatment strategies. This means… "See Your Doctor."

No information contained herein, as expressed, or as implied, or as might be interpreted by the reader, is intended to diagnose, treat, cure, or prevent any disease. That is why the reader is advised again to seek his or her own personal professional medical consultation.

I have done my very best to ensure that the contents of this book are accurate. The information contained herein is based upon my own personal research and personal experience and while I believe it to be correct and accurate as based entirely upon my own research and experience, it cannot be guaranteed in any way to be correct and accurate. No warrantee or guarantee of any kind is stated, intended, expressed, or implied.

While the information provided and the opinions expressed in this book are believed to be accurate and are based on the best judgment of the author, readers who fail to consult with appropriate health care authorities assume ALL risk for ANY injury and for consequences of any kind.

Neither the author, nor the publisher, nor any person or persons associated with the writing, editing, publication, printing, or distribution of this book is liable for any errors, inaccuracies, or omissions. The reader assumes ALL responsibility for ANY actions taken and is repeatedly advised to seek appropriate professional medical consultation.

Neither the U.S. Food and Drug Administration (USFDA) nor the American Medical Association (AMA) have approved any of the materials contained, practices described, or information presented in this book. The author does however recommend that the USFDA, the AMA, medicine, big medicine, big drug and pharmaceutical companies, and big money finally admit to us the benefits of natural and herbal remedies, which can quickly and cost effectively save millions of our dollars and both prolong and save millions of our lives each year.

Acknowledgements

I do not believe that it would have been possible to write my three books without the thoughtful and persistent encouragement of my granddaughter, Holly Kubicki who graduated from The State University of New York College at Buffalo in 2007 with honors and is now a certified secondary school Mathematics teacher in New York. She presently has her Masters Degree and, along with all of my children and grandchildren, has made us very proud.

Holly caused me to realize that my lifetime accumulation of health and fitness knowledge should be shared with others so that they too might benefit from all of the things that have contributed to my longevity, good health, and happiness. She was instrumental in the preparation of the early drafts of the manuscripts, which have now become this series of three books.

THOMAS TASSEFF

I have been very fortunate while writing all three of my books to have such a friend as Steven J. Wamback who did the technical and manual editing of later versions of the manuscripts and skillfully guided their progress toward publication and greater public appeal. Steve is a biologist, geologist, environmental scientist, and science writer who has managed numerous investigative and editorial projects in the natural sciences, public education, and biomedical research. Google: "Steven J. Wamback"

Chapter 1
Our Body is a Precision Electronic Machine

Our God-given body is a finely tuned machine with the unique ability to replicate and rejuvenate itself, to stay young and strong, and to last indefinitely. Of course, this simple fundamental principle has its basis in the assumption that we have provided the right conditions and have taken good care of ourselves.

Even though our body is composed largely of flesh and bone, it resembles a precision electronic machine in many ways. It runs on its own self-made electricity, without which the body cannot function. We essentially have a network of first class electrical circuitry running throughout our entire body. This internal "wiring" connects all of our cells and tissues while it orchestrates their precision life-preserving communication and functioning.

Bioelectricity is responsible for the operation of every system in our body including such functions as numerous and as diverse as physical movement, heartbeat, breathing, sensing pleasure or pain, speaking, hearing, dreaming, seeing, walking, running, sleeping, and thinking.

Specialized groups of cells carry out each of these various activities and functions; but they all depend upon adequate chemical nutrition, including properly balanced electrolytes, minerals, vitamins, metabolites, oxygen, and water, in order to maintain the optimal functioning of our complex electrical circuitry and of our entire body.

This finely tuned electrical network allows our cells to communicate with each other while organizing and directing all of life's tasks that our body performs…but again, only if we take good care of our body and provide it with all of the right nutritional and environmental conditions.

Ideal environmental conditions no longer actually exist in our natural world today as they once did. Therefore, we must find alternative ways to get rid of the dangerous toxins, which act as roadblocks, preventing many of the necessary nutrients from flowing freely to all of our cells. Nutrients and metabolites from our food, water, and air, feed our cellular circuitry and allow all of our cells to operate at their optimum metabolic efficiencies.

When properly functioning at their optimum efficiency, our cells communicate effectively with each other. This cellular communication allows cells to both replicate and rejuvenate themselves throughout our body while eliminating disease and the proliferation of any abnormal cells, which ultimately and effectively keeps us from aging or at least substantially slows down our aging process.

With the aging process slowed down or even reversed, our body and our cells are much more capable of winning the endless battle against yeast, fungus, virus, bacteria, parasites, and a whole host of toxins. Thus, keeping cells operating at their optimum efficiency for maintaining ideal health and maximum vitality is a potential "Fountain of Youth".

The aging process is responsible for the wasting of precious water, energy, electrolytes, and fluids from our cells, which leads to cell death without any cellular replacement. Senescence is the ending of a particular cell line and apoptosis is the programmed death of individual cells.

These are the specific causes of aging and old age at the cellular level. Another tragic alternative for old worn out undernourished cells is just the opposite of senescence and apoptosis: the rapid and abnormal overgrowth of cells via a whole series of pathological conditions collectively known as... Cancer.

When we have nourished our cells thoroughly and properly with the necessary hydrating minerals, lots of fresh air, and generous amounts of water, we easily flush our accumulated toxins away. This, in turn, initiates better nutrition, improves cellular energy-production, and favors greater intercellular communication, leading to growth and repair of cells, which is just one of the many self-sustaining cycles in our self-sustaining body.

When our body enjoys proper hydration, nutrition, and oxygenation, it becomes less acidic and the flow of nutrients to all of our cells is improved. Without proper hydration, nutrition, and oxygenation, our natural defenses are much more vulnerable to disease and to the effects of aging.

Healthy well-nourished cells (even old ones) have a better chance of surviving longer without leading to cellular senescence, apoptosis, or cancer. Healthy well-nourished cells have improved abilities for normal cellular growth, survival, reproduction, and repair.

Our body is composed of between 70 and 100 trillion cells, which ideally receive water, oxygen, and nourishment through 75,000 miles of arteries, veins, arterioles, vessels, micro vessels and capillaries. About 25 percent of the cells in the human body are red blood cells... also known as red blood corpuscles. The other 75 percent are white blood cells and comprise the body's immune system.

Red blood corpuscles are the free flowing red blood cells moving in our blood. The red blood cells in our blood contain molecules of the iron-based oxygen-transporting molecule hemoglobin. Hemoglobin's job is to take oxygen from our lungs, and deliver it to the rest of the cells in our body.

Our hearts pump our blood (and all it contains) throughout our body's tissues via blood flow through the whole circulatory system about once every 20 seconds. Oxygen diffuses into our cells while our blood is squeezed through the body's miles and miles of capillaries.

Hemoglobin also carries some of the wastes such as excess water and carbon dioxide back from our tissues, to the pulmonary capillaries in our alveoli (air sacs) in our lungs, where CO_2 and H_2O vapor are finally excreted via the exhaling half-portion of our breathing cycle.

Red blood cells are made in the bone marrow. Our white blood cells are also created in the bone marrow and transported to their major sites of activity where the majority of their duties take place as they leave our blood circulation to enter our body's tissues. Each of our various kinds of blood cells has differing life spans. Red blood cells last about 120 days in our bloodstream.

Our immune system produces several types of white cells, which each have distinct functions along with many characteristics in common, for fighting various infections and other assaults upon our body.

Neutrophil cells are the most important and most abundant of the white cells in our immune system. Also made in our bone marrow, neutrophils continuously circulate throughout our blood stream. They defend us against bacterial and fungal infections by moving into the infected tissue and attacking it via their production of hydrogen peroxide, which is a powerful anti-bacterial agent.

Hydrogen peroxide liberates free molecular oxygen, which is unstable and is therefore very reactive. This free oxygen may be considered a free radical because it eliminates the pathogens in our body by oxidizing them on contact. Our body creates these oxygen free radicals on its own for its own protection.

Eosinophil cells fight the infections caused by parasites. A parasitic infection is indicated when the eosinophil cell count is high. This cell type also reacts with substances that cause allergic reactions.

Basophil cells release histamines and initiate allergic reactions by releasing more histamines leading to inflammation. Inflammation is the natural response of our immune system to various types of physical or mental stresses and it attacks the various pathogens.

Inflammation is our body's attempt to remove these types of stress with a rise in temperature, an increase of blood flow, and delivery of the immune cells that fight off infections within injured tissues.

Lymphocyte cells are mostly responsible for providing our body with immunity. Lymphocytes achieve this by creating and releasing antibodies that bind themselves to pathogens (invaders in our body) and enable their destruction.

Monocyte cells are the cleanup crew that actually ingests the dead cells, tissue debris, old blood cells and anything that is left after an infectious agent has been killed or destroyed.

If we were to compare the size of any of our cells to a grain of sand, most of our cells are 25,000 times smaller than that grain of sand.

As you might recall from your high school and college introductory Biology courses, our cells contain organelles (mini organs) called mitochondria. (The term "mitochondria" is the plural form of the singular form mitochondrion.)

These mitochondria are the "powerhouses of our cells" where food nutrients, such as glucose, are metabolized and the energy produced is then stored in the three high-energy phosphate bonds of a molecule called adenosine triphosphate (ATP), which is known as "the energy currency of our cells".

British scientist, Dr. Peter D. Mitchell, won the Nobel Prize in 1978 for his contribution to the understanding of biological energy transfer, which ultimately led to the discovery of the body's anti-aging process. He elucidated the characteristics and functions of mitochondria as the main energy production units inside each of our cells as well in the cells of practically all living things.

Simplistically, mitochondrial powerhouses might be thought of as batteries or the cell's energy factories because they metabolize food and store the energy liberated from nutrients in the form of ATP (adenosine triphosphate).

Mitochondria are responsible for converting fats, sugars, and amino acids into energy, which gets stored in the form of the three high-energy phosphate bonds in ATP molecules.

THE OXYGEN LEGACY

Do you remember grudgingly studying (or even memorizing) the "Krebs Cycle" in school? This is merely a chemical chain reaction in which the energy of each molecule of glucose, through a series of intermediary biochemical steps, and is ultimately converted into 36 molecules of ATP... the main "energy currency" in the cells of all living things.

The breaking of the three high-energy-storage phosphate bonds in each ATP molecule releases the stored-up energy needed to run each of our body's 70 to 100 trillion cells and which sustains or powers life in practically all animals, plants, bacteria, protists, and fungi.

Our tissue cells contain various numbers of mitochondria within them depending upon their varying energy requirements. Some of our low-energy and less active body tissues may have as few as one or two mitochondria in each cell.

Our quite-active bicep muscles may have as many as 200 mitochondria in each cell. Our perpetually busy heart tissue cells have as many as 5,000 mitochondria each. Since our brains never stop working, even when we are asleep, brain cells also have thousands of mitochondria in each cell.

The more actively busy a cell is, the greater its energy requirements, and the more mitochondria it will have to convert the energy of glucose and other nutrient molecules into the high-energy phosphate bonds of ATP.

In order for us to survive, all of our cells must be fed with appropriate concentrations of all the necessary nutrients. Food is digested (broken down) in our digestive system by our digestive processes. With the help of stomach acids and enzymes, fats become fatty acids and glycerol; proteins become amino acids; and carbohydrates become simple sugars such as glucose.

Food nutrients liberated by digestion enter our bloodstream via tiny finger-like projections called villi in walls of the small intestine. Nutrients are absorbed via the capillary-rich villi and are then transferred to all of our 100 trillion cells via the blood and the circulatory system. The 75,000 miles of our circulatory system consists of its main pump... our beating heart, arteries, arterioles, veins, venules, microscopic capillaries, and blood.

The principal nutrient that our cells need is oxygen; and they cannot survive very long without receiving at least 60 percent of their optimum oxygen requirement.

If our body receives less than 60 percent of its required oxygen, our cells in turn receive less than they need which means that the cells with larger mitochondria and those with more mitochondria tend to suffer most because their energy demands are greatest.

Nutrients from food are metabolized in the cellular

mitochondria and are synthesized into energy-rich ATP molecules. Oxygen deficiency decreases the production of these energy-storing and energy-liberating ATP molecules and ultimately leads to abnormal, dead, or dying cells.

In order for us to remain healthy, every cell in our body must be continuously supplied with its proper nutrients and with its optimal amount of required oxygen. When our body is deprived of its much-needed oxygen, all of our body's physical and chemical processes are impaired.

If we suffer a continued deficit in our optimal oxygen requirements, carbon dioxide quickly accumulates in our blood. Excess CO_2 leads to acidic and anaerobic conditions, which cannot be easily reversed and which favors a host of diseases.

Oxygen deficiency weakens our immune system by deoxidizing it, thereby allowing the invasion of various pathogens and the spread of disease. A weakened immune system favors the proliferation of pathogens, toxins, and abnormal cell types. Pathogens, toxins, and abnormal cells take up residence in this anaerobic (oxygen-deficient) and acidic environment, which, under a suppressed or deficient immune system, is the only place where they can exist.

One of oxygen's main functions in our body is to serve as a blotter for soaking up extraneous and acidic protons or hydrogen (+1) ions. Every atom of oxygen is capable of picking up two acidic hydrogen ions and neutralizing them by forming H_2O ... water. Excess water is expelled from our bodies by exhalation, sweating, and urination along with other dissolved and excess compounds such as carbon dioxide, salts, and urea.

Both hydrogen ions and carbon dioxide molecules acidify our bodies and our blood. Pathogens and cancer cells are favored in acidic oxygen-poor environments. By optimizing our oxygen intake, uptake, and utilization, we can eliminate the acidic and anaerobic conditions that favor the proliferation of both pathogens and cancer cells.

Since we all have some degree of control over how much oxygen gets into our bodies, such as through aerobic exercise, deep breathing exercises, and using good nutrition and nutritional supplements to enhance oxygen delivery, we thus have some degree of control over the effects that pathogenic diseases, cancer, and old age might have on us. When it comes to disease, cancer, and aging, WE are in control.

Chapter 2
Antioxidants and Free Radicals

Mitochondria are the energy powerhouses of our cells. They slow down their energy production as we age, a result of the constant and fierce attacks by free radicals also known as oxidants. The immune system's cellular defense system becomes overwhelmed by excessive oxidative (free radical) assaults from the environment and can cause serious injury to our cells.

As we age, our bodies will lose 25% to 50% of our energy-capturing ability. If we don't do anything to recharge our system, we will always feel fatigue and lack of energy. This unfortunate result is due to the aging and subsequent lowered energy production of our mini energy factories, our mitochondria, which are deep in our cells and which produce less energy than when we were younger.

By raising the levels of antioxidants in our bloodstream, we can rid ourselves of the free radicals that rob us of energy, and which accelerate our aging process. When antioxidants enter the mitochondria of our cells, the resulting process floods our body with new energy. It does this by neutralizing any free radicals within our cells thereby fighting the aging process and increasing our cellular energy production.

When we acquire and retain too many free radicals, they are a form of internal pollution within our cells and lead to decreases in our energy levels as well as to a greater susceptibility to both infectious and non-infectious diseases.

Wherever free radicals occur, they act as pathogens within our bodies. Some of their sources include yeasts and other fungi, bacteria, parasites, viruses, and a myriad of other invading organisms and toxins that just do not belong in our body.

Presently, our world and consequently our bodies are under attack by many thousands of free radicals. They are in our polluted air and water, in plastics, and in many thousands of chemicals that enter our body every day. Free radicals are unstable because their atoms are missing an electron and they are looking for another electron to steal by bonding to anything they can.

THE OXYGEN LEGACY

Free radicals often chemically steal away electrons from just about any molecule in any cell they can contact within our heart, liver, lungs, brain, or any other vulnerable place in our body. Our body's normal and usual defense mechanisms can often become overburdened and we eventually can no longer defend ourselves from this pervasive and relentless free radical attack.

When free radicals attack our healthy cells, they often die. The death of our healthy cells causes illness, accelerated aging, and ultimately death. In order to destroy free radicals before they can harm us, it would be wise for us to take antioxidant supplements in addition to eating antioxidant-rich foods. An antioxidant-rich diet along with antioxidant supplements can help us to stay healthy and will prevent us from growing old before our time.

Our cell membranes need to remain continuously flexible to allow much-needed nutrients to enter into our cells and then into our mitochondria and thereby increase mitochondrial energy production. As we age, the amount of energy processed by our mitochondria decreases rather substantially. Considerable damage can be caused to the membranes of our mitochondria if free radicals aren't neutralized by antioxidants.

Free radicals create oxidative stress, which helps weaken our cells' ability to convert food to energy. As a result, this cellular damage makes us feel tired and initiates some of the first signs of aging by making us both look and feel older.

Free radicals are the main culprit in cell decomposition, thereby cumulatively resulting in our aging process. As we continue aging, more free radicals attack every cell in our body at a rate of approximately 100,000 times each day.

When high concentrations of free radicals attack our cells, the process is referred to as oxidative stress. Oxidative stress leads to the production of chemicals that create the oxidative damage. Free radicals only need a nanosecond to wreak their havoc, which is just enough time to do some cellular damage. Since there are millions of free radicals coursing through our bodies, they start snowballing the process of increasing oxidative damage.

With time, our total oxidative stress only worsens. This cellular destruction can be seen by the appearance of visible aging, with damaged skin, deep wrinkles, and loss of tone in our skin and that glow of youthfulness as the signs of aging are accelerated.

During the past several years, many articles have been written contending that free radicals are responsible for all disease and for premature aging. Although substantially correct, these researchers did not realize that our bodies actually create some oxygen free radicals in our own immune systems, which are used to destroy yeasts, viruses, fungi, toxins, harmful bacteria, parasites, and other pathogens.

The immune system's white blood cells are responsible for making hydrogen peroxide and use it to oxidize all of the offending pathogens and toxins.

Our body's ability to produce hydrogen peroxide (H_2O_2) in our own immune system is essential for life and good health. It neither is a toxin nor is it necessarily an undesirable by-product.

Hydrogen peroxide is relatively unstable and breaks down into water and unstable atoms of oxygen, which are highly reactive. By delivering extra oxygen, hydrogen peroxide oxidizes many of the body's pathogens on contact, since they cannot survive in an oxygen rich environment.

We are constantly under attack by thousands of other types of free radicals from our polluted air, from water pollution, from plastics, and from thousands of chemicals and toxins that make their way into our bodies every day.

Our body is constantly being overwhelmed and just does not have the complete defensive power that is necessary to fight off these attacks with our natural compliment of oxygen free radicals that are naturally produced by our body's immune system.

As our cells get thicker and more rigid with age, it becomes more difficult for oxygen and other nutrients to enter them. Chronic tension and stress (both physical and emotional) make our cell walls deteriorate faster thereby making us more vulnerable to many age related disorders.

The Life Extension Foundation purports that when Acetyl-L-Carnitine enters our blood stream it penetrates the cell walls very effectively. The presence of Alpha lipoic acid destroys potentially harmful free radicals and invigorates antioxidants.

Antioxidants are the best supplements that we can take to prevent the speeding up of our aging process. Antioxidants slow our aging process down by eliminating the free radicals before they can damage the healthy cells in our body.

The ORAC test is a measurement of antioxidant potential of the foods we eat. This test measures the "Oxygen Radical Absorbance Capacity" of various foods and supplements, by evaluating their oxygen radical absorbance capacity. As the antioxidant-containing foods and supplements achieve a higher rating on the ORAC test, the better it is for us in eliminating free radicals and disease.

Glutathione is recognized as being the most powerful antioxidant for our body for fighting off aging, boosting our immune system, and for building energy and strength. It also helps reactivate and maintain the activity of other important antioxidants, such as Vitamin C and Vitamin E, and keeps them working.

Our body fluids and every cell in our body contain glutathione, which cleanses our liver, kidneys, lungs, and intestines by helping to detoxify the chemicals and pollutants that we inhale, ingest or produce within our body.

Glutathione is a very simple molecular substance that is continuously produced in our body. It is a tri-peptide, which consists of three of the twenty or so simple building blocks of protein (amino-acids) including glutamate, cysteine, and glycine, and which can be ingested by the body through both foods and supplements.

Glutathione also contains a very sticky atom of sulfur, which acts like fly paper. All of the free radicals and toxins such as mercury and other heavy metals stick to it. Therefore, glutathione is one of the most critical components of our detoxification system because all toxins stick to it. These are then carried into the bile and stool to be eliminated from our body.

Glutathione is the most important of all the antioxidants,

and it easily might be considered the "Mother of All Antioxidants". It shows great promise in the prevention of heart disease, cancer, dementia, and aging. Glutathione is essential in the treatment of both autism and Alzheimer's disease.

Pollution, toxins, poor diet, stress, trauma, infections, medications, and various forms of radiation deplete our body of its glutathione. As a result, our liver eventually becomes overloaded and damaged, which makes it unable to do an efficient job of detoxification.

Glutathione deficiencies have been found in people with heart disease, assorted cancers, chronic fatigue syndrome, chronic infections, diabetes, Alzheimer's disease, autoimmune disease, arthritis, autism, Parkinson's disease, liver disease, kidney problems, and a host of others. Therefore, we should improve our ability to maintain a high level of glutathione, since it is critical for recovery from nearly all chronic illnesses.

When our body's toxic load becomes too great, problems occur, which overwhelm us with too much oxidative stress or too many toxins. Glutathione then becomes depleted, which leaves us unable to protect ourselves from free radicals, infections, and cancer, by the neutralization and elimination of toxins. This leads us into a downward spiral of chronic illness and further disease.

Glutathione has a critical function in recycling valuable antioxidants. The free radicals are passed around from Vitamin C to Vitamin E to lipoic acid and finally to glutathione, in order to manage the free radicals and to recycle other antioxidants. Soon after this, the body can either reduce or regenerate more protective glutathione molecules as needed.

There are genes in our DNA that code for the production of specific enzymes, which allow the body to create and recycle glutathione in the body. These genes have been identified as GSTM1, GSTP1 to mention just a few.

Nearly all very sick people are missing this genetic function and consequently, its beneficial potential. One third of our population suffers from chronic disease, which is attributed to the limited function or absence of these glutathione-production genes. This results in an inadequate production or no production of glutathione thereby causing their glutathione-deficient bodies to break down, to age rapidly, and to become extremely ill.

By keeping our glutathione levels high, we stay healthy, boost our performance, age well, and prevent disease. Glutathione is the body's main antioxidant and detoxifier. It is critical to the immune system by controlling inflammation, protecting our cells, and helping our energy metabolism processes to run well.

Glutathione also helps us to reach our peaks in both physical and mental functioning. By raising glutathione levels in our body, we reduce recovery time, decrease muscle damage, increase strength and endurance, and shift fat metabolism to lean muscle development.

The human species evolved long before 80,000 toxic industrial chemicals were introduced into our world. These chemical toxins are now found in every corner of our environment. We evolved long before man-made electromagnetic radiation appeared everywhere. Our species arose prior to the pollution of our skies, lakes, and oceans and long before our teeth were filled with amalgam fillings comprised of mercury and lead.

This is why throughout the ages most people survived with only the basic version of the genetic detoxification software that was encoded in our DNA but which is only mediocre at ridding the body of our modern day toxins in the modern world.

It just so happens that we did not need any greater protection when we humans first evolved. No one knew that we would one day be polluting our planet, poisoning ourselves, and eating an over processed additive enhanced, but nutrient-depleted diet thousands of years later.

Since most of us didn't require any such additional genetic

software, almost half of our present population has a limited capacity to get rid of toxins. This happens because people are missing the GSTM-1 functional gene. It is one of the most important genes needed in the process of creating and recycling glutathione in the body.

However, we can do a number of things to increase glutathione levels in our body and afford ourselves the necessary level of protection that evolution has not caught up with yet.

Methods to Optimize Our Glutathione Levels and to Live a Longer, Happier, and Healthier Life

- Eat sulfur-rich foods such as onions, garlic, cabbage, cauliflower, broccoli, kale, and collards. All of these should be included in our diets.

- Consume Bioactive Whey Protein as it contains cysteine and other amino acid building blocks for synthesis of glutathione.

- Take N-acetyl-cysteine, which has always been used to treat asthma, lung disease, and liver failure.

- Supplement Alpha Lipoic acid in our diet. This nutrient is almost as important as glutathione in our cells for energy production, blood-sugar control, brain health, and detoxification. It is usually made in our body, but often becomes depleted due to all of our stresses.

- Take Selenium supplements, as this mineral is important in helping our body to recycle and produce more glutathione.

- Take Milk Thistle (silymarin). Milk Thistle has been used in treating liver disease and helps increase levels of glutathione.

- Take Vitamins C and E. They work together and help to recycle glutathione.

- Take Folate, Vitamin B-6, and Vitamin B-12. They are important coenzymes involved in the biochemical process of our body's production of glutathione.

- Get more exercise. Exercise boosts our glutathione levels, which also boosts our immune system, improves detoxification, and helps increase our body's antioxidants. Exercise does not have to be physically hard; it could be walking or jogging.

- Take Dr. Stephen Langer's Precursor Complex and Bioactive Whey Protein. It is "Certified Organic" UN-denatured Bioactive Whey Protein. It boosts glutathione by giving the body pure, high quality, bio-available protein to make its own glutathione.

By being un-denatured, it means that whey protein is processed under low temperatures, which maintains its delicate amino acid structures that our body needs for producing glutathione.

Many other proteins are denatured during processes where they are heat processed and pasteurized, which break down the native proteins and do nothing to boost or preserve the desired glutathione proteins.

Whey protein nutritional supplements can be blended with fruits and milk or juices to make a healthy glutathione-enhancing and thereby life-saving protein shake or smoothie.

Chapter 3
Astaxanthin: The Alpha Antioxidant

Astaxanthin is a member of the carotenoid family and has been proclaimed as the most powerful antioxidant. It comes from deep-red-colored micro algae that are naturally grown in fresh water and which has the ability to live for long periods of time.

Astaxanthin has miraculous power with its unique ability to protect itself from oxidation, UV radiation, and a multitude of other environmental stresses. After it is harvested and concentrated, it is recognized as the most powerful anti-oxidant in the world.

Astaxanthin is a powerful new medical breakthrough, which shows its power in its ability to keep our hearts pumping powerfully; and it is about 500 times more beneficial to the heart than Vitamin-E. It does a terrific job in eliminating inflammation of the heart; it keeps our vision clear, it keeps our brains healthy, and still, it does much more.

Many doctors believe that astaxanthin should be regarded as the natural miracle of the 21st Century and it is really an anti-aging miracle, which we can all afford.

Research has demonstrated that astaxanthin is ten times stronger in scavenging free radicals than carotenoids such as lutein, zeaxanthin, and beta-carotene; and it is one hundred times stronger than alpha tocopherol. Astaxanthin's benefits have been published on television, in the news, in magazines, in books, and in medical journals.

Astaxanthin is a small molecule that can easily cross the blood-brain and retina-brain barriers. Due to its antioxidant activities and its permeability of the blood-brain barrier and retina-brain barriers, it has benefits for the inflammations caused by diabetes, cardio vascular disease, vision problems, and a number of neurological conditions.

Astaxanthin protects the cellular and mitochondrial membranes as well as ocular (eye) tissues from further oxidative damage and helps them in their restoration processes. It promotes excellent short-term memory by crossing the blood-brain barrier, which is composed of very tightly woven microscopic cells around the capillaries that lead into our brains. This barrier is designed to keep bacteria, viruses, and other pathogens from harming the brain.

Antioxidants are either water-soluble or fat-soluble, which limits them to travel to separate and specific areas of the body in order to destroy any invading free radicals. However, astaxanthin is considered an alpha antioxidant because it is both water-soluble and fat-soluble, which means it can pretty much go where it pleases... even across the blood brain barrier.

After it enters the brain, astaxanthin destroys every free radical with which it comes in contact. Animal studies have shown that astaxanthin lowers inflammation markers and promotes excellent short-term memory retention.

With its miraculous power for destroying just about any free radicals, astaxanthin is one of a few limited substances that can cross the blood-brain barrier.

Astaxanthin is very important to our brain's development by raising its DHA and EPA fatty acids that are essential in building a strong, healthy and efficient brain. DHA and EFA lower triglycerides levels, which helps protect the heart. Astaxanthin also helps the brain as demonstrated by improved cognitive functioning.

Astaxanthin also helps improve our immune system, thyroid function, skin health, bone health, blood sugar control, liver health, joint health, blood detoxification, and cholesterol.

Everyone should supplement their diets with extracts, concentrates, capsules, and suspensions of this miraculous nutrient and lifesaving algae-based antioxidant.

Chapter 4
Our Links to Aging

Research indicates that our nervous systems are just as old as we are. Brain cells and neurons are very sensitive to environmental and oxidative stresses. They are not generally very easily replaced; so, protection and conservation of these vital components is of utmost importance.

Recent studies have shown that our cells "wiring" needs to remain consistent throughout our lifespan. The most common problems related to aging are linked directly to the degeneration of the nervous system. This means various parts of our body age more, and more rapidly, than others.

Even though we may not be able to stop entirely the aging

process, we can take specific preventative actions, which slow this process to effectively prevent and delay some of the most pervasive and debilitating problems associated with aging.

We had more brain cells when we were born than we ever will have at any point in our future lives.

Parkinson's disease and Alzheimer's disease are two of the most common neurological disorders and are linked to a lack of nerve tissue development. Even though some neurological degeneration is a natural part of life, this gradual nerve degeneration process can be slowed down and thereby minimize the ill effects on our overall health.

Four of the most common age-related complaints are:

- Lack of energy;

- Brain dysfunction such as mental fatigue, depression and inability to concentrate;

- Diabetes;

- Digestive disorders.

Although these are all common age-related complaints due to neurological degeneration, it doesn't mean that they should be considered normal or inevitable. As we get older, we may notice that many people appear to be suffering from a particular ailment or disease that we believe from which we too will eventually suffer. This prophecy and this belief do not necessarily have to come true.

Degeneration of our minds and nervous systems is not a fate entirely cast in stone. Much of our potential neurological degeneration is a result of bad habits, risky lifestyles, and bad diets. We can still prevent many of these degenerative processes by actively making healthy choices now. In some cases, we can even reverse some of the negative effects of a lifetime of making bad choices.

All of our body's energy is produced by the conversion of food and nutritional energy in the mitochondria of our cells. As we mentioned previously, mitochondria are infinitesimally tiny structures located in practically every one of our cells. They are the "energy furnaces" responsible for cellular energy production throughout our entire body. The optimum functioning of these energy "powerhouses" within each of our cells relates directly to our overall health and vitality.

Since our body's energy flow is controlled by our mitochondria, they must receive their optimum amounts of the proper nutrients. The term "respiration" is often confused with the process of "breathing". Breathing is merely the taking in of air from the environment into our lungs so that oxygen can enter while carbon dioxide and water vapor can exit our bloodstreams.

Respiration is actually the process of converting food and nutritional energy into forms readily usable by our cells. Respiration is chemically the opposite of photosynthesis in plants. Photosynthesis is the means by which green plants capture energy from the Sun, along with water and carbon dioxide, synthesize, and store that energy in the form of glucose.

Conversely, respiration is the chemical metabolism of glucose and other nutrients, in the presence of oxygen to liberate energy and store it in the form of the high-energy phosphate bonds of adenosine triphosphate (ATP). Remember… ATP is the energy currency of our cells. Carbon dioxide and water are the waste products of aerobic respiration.

All of this energy metabolism and energy conversion (via the dreaded Krebs Cycle) takes place within our mitochondria. That is why mitochondria are known as "the powerhouses of our cells".

Mitochondria are adversely affected by any of the free radicals to which they have been exposed. Mitochondrial damage can be caused through their exposure to toxins,

THE OXYGEN LEGACY

heavy metals, drugs, electro-magnetic pollution, yeasts, viruses, bacteria, parasites and a host of other pathogens and toxin in our every-day lives.

Different types of body tissues have cells with varying numbers of mitochondria (singular: mitochondrion) in each type of tissue and cells. As we have mentioned previously, the number of mitochondria in each type of cell depends upon the type of tissue and its specific need for energy.

Our "busiest" and most active cells such as heart, muscle, and brain cells have the greatest number of mitochondria per cell. Less-busy cells such as epithelium and glandular cells have many fewer mitochondria.

Some tissue types have as few as one mitochondrion per cell. Since our constantly beating heart muscle cells have very high metabolic rates, and hence very high energy-requirements, they each may contain 5,000 or more mitochondria.

At conception, all of our mitochondria come from the egg cells produced and contributed by our mothers. The mitochondria from our fathers' sperm cells do not become incorporated into the offspring. Mitochondria have their own DNA, which is separate from our chromosomal DNA in the cell nucleus; and it more closely resembles the DNA in bacterial cells.

Our chromosomal DNA is acquired from both of our parents but our mitochondrial DNA comes only from our mothers. That is why both geneticists and genealogists use mitochondrial DNA to trace genetic lineages, but again only from the line of mothers. If a woman has no daughters, sisters, or maternal aunts, her specific line of mitochondrial DNA ends forever.

Each mitochondrion contains about 3,000 genes. Only about three percent of these genes are related directly to energy production while 95 percent of them are responsible for other diverse and specialized functions such as growth, repair, and reproduction of the mitochondria themselves.

The energy captured and converted in our mitochondria by the process of cellular respiration is responsible for all of the energy-requiring and energy-using processes that take place within us as well as in most other living things.

The mitochondria, the small energy furnaces that reside in every one of our body's cells, use fuel that comes from the food we eat and the oxygen in the air we breathe, which is needed to burn that food in order to obtain the fuel. This process produces the necessary heat for the body.

Bioluminescent light (as seen in fireflies) is also produced from the energy released from adenosine triphosphate (ATP). ATP is much like a rechargeable battery in that it can be transported anywhere in the body for various purposes. The waste products of oxygen free radicals and toxins can clog and damage parts of the cell, such as the mitochondrial DNA, which is the blueprint for creating more mitochondria within our cells.

The mitochondria in every cell and the nucleus in every cell each contain their own separate DNA. When the mitochondria of any of our body's cells fail to obtain their optimum amount of needed energy, they become damaged and our energy flow decreases and deteriorates all of the cells through our body.

This can lead to just about any type of disease since all diseases are linked to faulty mitochondrial metabolism resulting in neurodegenerative diseases. Symptoms of these problems, as well as *which* disease occurs, depends upon the location of the mitochondria and the tissues they inhabit.

As an example, take a look at the skin on your hands because the skin cells replace themselves about every two weeks. Eventually, with the passing of time, our skin loses elasticity, becomes dry and has wrinkles. This is due to the constant bombardment of thousands of free radicals, which gradually result in damage to the DNA of the mitochondria, which causes mutations that are responsible for the loss of quality in production of our collagen.

During a study performed on a 90-year-old man, it was revealed that his mitochondria were damaged in 95 percent of his muscular tissue, while in a 5-year-old there was no damage at all. Mitochondrial DNA obviously develops mutations as we age, due to the constant bombardment of pathogens and free radicals.

Many more of our body's cells are also affected by free radicals and cause mutations of our cells in a similar manner. Inherited or spontaneous mutations of DNA can cause mitochondrial-related diseases, which can develop into almost endless problems.

Researchers have barely begun to link health problems to mitochondrial dysfunction. It is known that all individuals who suffer from genetic mitochondrial diseases are energy-deficient and complain of chronic pain, chronic fatigue, heart problems, kidney problems, and even other problems with other tissues or organs that require a lot of energy. Researchers are now seeing the same symptoms in our aging population.

When we do mentally challenging work and become easily fatigued, that is an indication that the mitochondria in the cells of our nervous system are inefficient and failing.

During our youthful school years, we were able to

concentrate and study in school for hours and memorize our lessons much better. As we got older, they all became more difficult and concentrating for any length of time can easily wear us out.

These are problems associated with aging but they are really symptoms of neurological degeneration and mitochondrial breakdown in the cells of our nervous system.

Glucose is a very important fuel used by all the cells of our body. Brain cells are constantly working and they use much more energy than most of our other cells. Almost half of our body's total energy supply is used by the brain and nervous system, which requires an uninterrupted supply of glucose because the nerve cells are unable to store glucose like any of our other cells. As that supply of glucose decreases, it reduces the necessary food for our brain cells, which began to die, thereby causing serious neurological disorders.

Our overall health and vitality are directly related to the health and vitality of our mitochondria. Our mitochondria are negatively affected by exposure to pathogens, free radicals, heavy metals, toxic chemicals, pharmaceutical drugs, and electric pollution, and many more pathogens, which are all in our every day lives of our modern world.

Thousands of studies have linked abnormal mitochondrial metabolism to neurodegenerative diseases such as: Parkinson's, Alzheimer's, diabetes, obesity, autoimmune problems, heart disease, stroke, cancer and more. At least 50 million people in the USA are affected with the conditions that involve mitochondrial dysfunction.

Our metabolic systems are not capable of managing excess nutrition such as the high fat, low fiber, high sugar, and over-processed foods in our modern diet. Our bodies are not designed to effectively deal with this modern diet, which has arisen since the industrial-agricultural revolution of the past 200 or so years.

Many of our foods should be considered as "junk foods" because they are made with over-processed, low-nutrient flour, excess fats, and simple sugars to make them tastier and supposedly to give us more energy.

Our cells are struggling to obtain sufficient quantities of the proper nutrients needed to stay healthy and for us to survive. This causes our cells to enter a starvation survival mode in which our nervous system receives messages that we are still hungry in an attempt to provide our cells with more nutrients.

When we consume excess quantities of food, the excess is nearly all converted to fat. Fats normally enter our mitochondrial powerhouses and are converted into our body's main energy currency molecule ATP (adenosine triphosphate) for cellular energy.

After we have consumed excessive quantities of high fats and sugars, our body has to transport the fat and burn via normal metabolic processes. Our body must also remove the sugars and convert them to glucose for cellular energy production in our mitochondrial energy factories.

This excess nutrition "confuses" our muscle and liver cells. Large quantities of partially burned fat molecules accumulate, get stored, and hinder the cellular removal of glucose from our blood stream. Glucose is normally converted to energy in our mitochondria but the excess leads to a breakdown in the normal metabolic machinery. This breakdown in normal metabolic functioning is known as metabolic syndrome.

The enzyme nutrient L-Carnitine is responsible for transporting fats to our mitochondria where fats are ultimately converted into energy. L-Carnitine is also used to carry away excess fat because fat interferes with mitochondrial metabolism and efficient energy production.

Researchers have shown that a deficiency of L-Carnitine is at least partially responsible for pre-diabetic conditions. A deficiency of L-Carnitine induces mitochondrial clogging by incompletely oxidized molecules while patient subjects on a diet supplemented with L-Carnitine were shown to have a healthy ratio of both partially oxidized and completely oxidized fats.

This means that a deficiency of L-Carnitine in a high fat diet induces a shortage of available L-Carnitine because much of it was being used to transport excess fat to the mitochondria while leaving very little L-Carnitine available to remove partially oxidized fats.

If partially oxidized fats are not removed, mitochondrial clogging occurs, which prevents the normal metabolism of glucose by the mitochondria and that can lead to some forms of diabetes. But by having sufficient L-Carnitine, excess fats and partially metabolized fats are removed from the mitochondria and hence, glucose metabolism is enhanced, yielding better and more efficient energy production at the mitochondria and lower blood sugar levels as mitochondria are free to do their job... efficiently metabolizing sugars.

It is very important to reduce unnecessary metals and toxins in our body because they can cause problems with our brain, our joints, and other parts of our body. Even if metals and toxins are successfully removed from the body, their residual damage remains and it must be repaired or more damage to our health will ensue.

THE OXYGEN LEGACY

We are capable of living a longer, healthier, happier, and more productive life by contributing essential nutrients to feed our mitochondria and help neutralize toxins that can cause our mitochondrial dysfunctions.

Some specific nutrients that could help to enhance our health and longevity by nurturing our mitochondria are:

- Alpha lipoic acid (ALA) destroys potentially harmful free radicals and increases the effectiveness of other antioxidants such as vitamins C and E by recharging these key antioxidants and keeping them in our body at least twice as long as normal. ALA also enables N-Acetyl-L-Cysteine to enter all of our cells more easily. Lead is the most deadly of all metals. Vitamins C and E are very effective and have always proven to protect our body from damage caused by free radicals.

- Acetyl- L-Carnitine makes it easier for alpha lipoic acid (ALA) to enter our cells' mitochondria and it allows them to receive all of their necessary nutrients, thereby preventing dysfunctional mitochondrial metabolism (Metabolism Syndrome), which is necessary in preventing and eliminating nearly all forms of disease.

- N-Acetyl-L-Cysteine (NAC) protects our liver by

neutralizing metals and reducing exposure to toxins. NAC also helps our body to produce its own powerful antioxidant, glutathione. Glutathione is included in every one of our body's cells and helps boost immunity, fights free radicals within our cells and binds metals and toxins to be excreted from our body.

- Malic acid originates in apples and is the most effective for removal of aluminum from the body. Aluminum is another most harmful metal to our body, which does a great deal of damage to our brains and nerves. It causes poor nerve functioning, poor learning, poor memory, and diminished cognitive skills. Aluminum is almost impossible to avoid because it is included in vaccines as a preservative, antiperspirants, antacids, beverage cans and drinking water. Once aluminum enters our body, it was almost impossible to get rid of it until scientists discovered that malic acid removes it. Malic acid worked better than a treatment that was specifically manufactured to remove metals from the body. Hence, the old saying that, "An apple a day keeps the doctor away" has a genuine basis in biochemical fact!

- Vitamin B-5 (panthothenic acid) is an important nutrient and supplement that is needed to rejuvenate our adrenal glands by forming the key enzyme that creates Cortisol.

Cortisol is one of the best-known hormones produced by the adrenal glands and it serves to regulate our immune system. When the Adrenal glands are strong, they produce the necessary amount of cortisol and our immune system functions very well. When the adrenal glands are over-stressed, they become fatigued and result in a plummeting amount of cortisol production.

Cortisol deficiency is very common and most unfortunate in our world today. Low cortisol concentrations cause the adrenal glands to continue producing more stress hormones. This might continue for years, which finally exhausts the adrenals.

This is one of the main reasons that more and more people are afflicted with allergies. We experience a myriad of problems when the body makes either too little or too much cortisol.

Low cortisol levels result in a weakened immune system. By having less cortisol, our immune system becomes overactive and releases histamines and other inflammatory substances that cause allergic symptoms.

In over 90 percent of allergy cases, the fatigue of our

adrenals is not permanent. We can strengthen our adrenals and give them a chance to rest and rebuild with the following supplements:

- Panthothenic acid (vitamin B-5), 500 mg can be taken twice a day… once in the morning and once at 2:00 PM because of the adrenals rhythmic function of high activity in the morning and afternoon then slowing down in the evening.

- Licorice herb (Licorice Root) helps maintain healthy cortisol levels by preventing our liver from breaking down our produced cortisol. It was recommended to start with 1,500 mg. twice daily, then after a few weeks, decrease to 700-1000 mg twice per day.

- DHEA (dehydropiandrosterone) 10-25 mg. could be added. DHEA is the other major hormone made by the adrenals.

A proper amount of sleep and a good night's rest are very important because the longer we stay awake, our adrenals are forced to work overtime and this causes them to become even weaker.

We need to avoid high glycemic carbohydrates by staying away from any processed foods or foods that contain refined sugar or flour. These cause our bodies to secrete more insulin by causing our adrenals to work overtime and pumping out more cortisol to meet our high insulin levels, thereby causing tremendous stress on our adrenal glands (and our pancreas).

We should avoid stimulants like coffee because caffeine exhausts the adrenal glands. Ridding ourselves of caffeine addiction along with a general detoxification should be a big help.

Chapter 5
Discovery of an All-Natural Anti-Aging Formula

The aging process is happening everywhere throughout our universe from the stars, planets, other worlds, and in our own world, as we know it. No matter what we do, we cannot reverse time or even stop the aging process within our body.

We can minimize most of our potential health disorders by supplying our body with its necessary antioxidants and nutrients, thereby slowing the aging process and enabling us to live a longer, healthier, happier, and more productive life.

Natural substances that our body normally manufactures in

sufficient quantities for optimum health during our youth gradually decrease with age. This means that the mitochondria, the main energy generators within our cells, began to decay after about 25 years, which accelerated the aging process. Therefore, we can slow down the aging process through improved mitochondrial health by supplementing our body with required antioxidants in our diet and via nutritional supplements.

Every day of our lives, our cells feel the effects of normal aging and we should take the necessary steps at any time to maintain a healthy lifestyle by providing our cells with their necessary nutrients to function properly and protect them from free radical damage. Many of us are walking around with weak and dying mitochondria in our cells. This causes more of our cells to die prematurely.

There is a product that neutralizes free radicals 24 hours a day and continues 7 days a week by keeping a high level of antioxidants in our body and which helps protect our cells from oxidative damage. It improves our body's cellular performance by helping oxygen and other nutrients to enter our cells and nourish them. This helps convert food into energy and aids our immune system in creating more of its natural antioxidants, which ultimately destroys free radicals.

Two Noble Prize-winning Doctors, Dr. Bruce Ames and

Dr. Tory Hagen of the University of California, invented an all-natural anti-aging remedy. These two Noble Prize winners developed and patented a unique cell-enhancing formula. It was given the name "Juvenon" (U.S. Patent No. 5,916,912).

For many years, Dr. Ames and Dr. Hagen were taking their own patented combination every day: 1,000 mg of acetyl-L-carnitine (ALC), 300 mg of biotin, 154 mg of calcium and 117 mg of phosphorous to breathe additional energy into our cells. It helps to slow the aging process and actually reverses the aging process.

This regimen also gives our cells protection from roaming packs of free radicals that lower our cells' special miniature, energy-converting, ATP-producing, factories'... mitochondria... energy levels. These two doctors were able to slow down the aging process and make their bodies feel 15-20 years younger.

The above-mentioned proteins and minerals can reinforce our body's own free radical production and keep our cells fully charged for maximum cellular protection from free radicals. This miraculous accomplishment takes place by getting anti-oxidants directly into the mitochondria to fight the free radicals that are responsible for stealing our energy and speeding up our aging processes.

This means that we can keep our minds and memories at their peaks; and we can also enjoy improved concentration, as well as greatly improved energy levels, and we will remain looking young, when we are actively repairing and rejuvenating our cells by reducing and eliminating free radicals.

Placing antioxidants back into our body's cells liberates energy and stops free radicals from further attacking our cells and releasing the chemicals that speed up old age leading to the plethora of diseases that are associated with aging.

Chapter 6
Our Body and DNA

Our body has the miraculous ability to renew itself continually by removing damaged cells and replacing them with new ones. This renewal process allows our body to stay young and functional for many years.

This renewal process begins to slow down as we become older and our body no longer replaces the bad cells (dying and abnormal cells) at the same pace. This leads to the proliferation of more non-functional cells and thereby exacerbates the aging process and all the problems that come with it... such as cancer and Alzheimer's disease to name just a few.

Recent research indicates that some of our body's renewal processes slow down and cellular division eventually stops entirely as we get older. This cessation in cellular division involves the telomeres in some of the genes contained in the DNA in the nuclei of our cells.

This calls for a brief introduction to DNA (deoxyribonucleic acid) and its normal and abnormal functioning within our cells. Our body is composed of 70 to 100 trillion cells and all have mitochondria, the energy powerhouses of our cells where nutrients and oxygen are converted to a usable form of energy, ATP.

Each one of our cells normally contains 23 pairs of chromosomes, for a combined total of 46 chromosomes. Half of them come from each of our parents and contain their respective contributions of DNA.

Each chromosome is an organized structure comprised of an organized coil of DNA and protein found in the nuclei of cells and each of which contains about 24,500 genes. Structurally, DNA is comparable to a spiral staircase or a twisted ladder with 24,500 steps or rungs. Each half of the ladder consists of long chains of the four nucleotides, A, G, T, and C.

DNA (deoxyribonucleic acid) contains and controls the genetic instructions in the development of all living organisms. In our body, DNA is the fundamental blueprint, for an individual's genetic makeup and a full genetic complement of DNA is contained in the nucleus of each of our cells.

The Human Genome Project has very nearly completed its work in identifying and elucidating the complete structure of the entire human genome and new discoveries are being made every day about this grand and complex blueprint, which defines who we are and where we came from in a number of biochemical, evolutionary, and genealogical perspectives.

DNA in a Nutshell

In this section, I shall briefly review everything the average layperson needs to know about DNA in an overly simplistic but thoroughly understandable analogy to a protein-making factory with a front office nucleus and a protein manufacturing assembly line process.

All life as we know it is based upon the structure and function of proteins, which are merely long chains of the twenty or so different amino acids.

Our bodies and all of our cells are largely composed of proteins in a physical and structural sense. Think of the protein Keratin, which comprises the physical structure (composition, shape, and form) of hair, nails, and skin cells. A similar protein, Chitin, composes the shells of insects and crustaceans. Another protein, Elastin, gives stretchability to our skin and connective tissues.

In addition to making up body structure, proteins also serve in biochemically functional ways such as hormones (like insulin) and enzymes (like pepsin), which initiate, carry out, and speed up the thousands of chemical reactions that take place in each of our cells and in each of our bodies. At its most simple and most fundamental level:

DNA is the blueprint for protein.

If we think of each cell as a sort of industrial park for the manufacture of protein and the nucleus as the main office in every cell, we will begin to understand how DNA works in the synthesis of protein.

When cells divide, so does their DNA in a process called replication. The DNA molecule "unzips" and then makes an exact replica of itself for each new cell. DNA replication during cell division is analogous to opening a new branch office and associated factory by ensuring that the new location has an exact copy of the blueprints for the final manufactured product... protein.

Each half of the twisted DNA ladder consists of long chains of the nucleotides A, G, C, and T on a sugar (deoxyribose) backbone. These stand for Adenine, Guanine, Cytocine,

THE OXYGEN LEGACY

and Thymine respectively. Thymine (T) is replaced by Uracil (U) in the RNA molecule.

Every three of these nucleotides in sequence is called a Codon and ultimately codes for one amino acid in the final protein molecule.

The complete list or chart of all 64 possible codon combinations (AAA, CAT, ACT, GGC, TTT, etc.) and their 20 associated amino acids, as well as a few stop and start codons, **IS** the Genetic Code, which even has many built-in failsafe mechanisms that MAY negate the effects of some mutations.

Several different combinations may code for the same amino acid thus reducing the effects of some mutations. There is sufficient overlap in the Genetic Code that some mutations might still result in the proper sequence of amino acids in the final protein product.

Mutations are merely wrong or missing nucleotides (AGTC) in the DNA sequence.

The assembly line for proteins lies outside of the nucleus in the cytoplasm of each cell. These assembly lines are the sites of protein synthesis called Ribosomes. In high school biology, we memorized the fact that, "Ribosomes are the sites of protein synthesis".

The cell's main office, the nucleus, sends out messages transcribed from the DNA blueprints for proteins in the form of its sister molecule RNA (ribonucleic acid). (Ribose and deoxyribose are simply sugar molecules in the long spiral backbone structure of RNA and DNA respectively.)

There are three kinds of RNA: (m, t, and r).

Messenger or mRNA is the transcribed message from the DNA in the main office or nucleus.

Like trucks and forklifts, Transfer RNA (tRNA) carries amino acids from nutrients to the ribosomal assembly lines.

Ribosomal RNA (rRNA) comprises the structure and function of the ribosomal assembly lines where the final proteins themselves are actually made.

DNA remains in the nucleus (the main office) and is transcribed into RNA from the DNA blueprint for sending out to the cytoplasm and to the ribosomes where proteins are rolled out like new cars off a Detroit assembly line.

Each 3-nucleotide unit of DNA, and hence of any transcribed RNA, called a codon, codes for one amino acid in the final protein molecule. Just like trucks bringing raw materials into a factory, tRNA brings in the amino acids to the ribosomes where the protein molecules are assembled according to the original DNA blueprint in the office and the mRNA message from the office.

There are also "Start and Stop" Codons in DNA and hence in RNA to help regulate the protein-making process by providing jumping-on and jumping-off points for the enzymes at the ribosomes, which like factory workers on an assembly line, perform all of the actual labor in assembling and adding the finishing touches to the protein final products.

This process of protein synthesis is called Translation because the original blueprint from DNA is ultimately translated into the final product... Protein molecules. That is what makes each of us different in both the physical and the genetic sense. Differences in our genetic makeup, our DNA, ultimately lead to differences in our Proteins.

Making Protein is What DNA is all About.

Table-1 demonstrates an analogous comparison between a factory setting manufacturing process and the cellular synthesis of proteins as a means for understanding DNA, RNA, and their functions in living things.

The DNA Factory-Office-Assembly-Line Analogy

Manufacturing Concept	Biological Equivalent
Products Manufactured	Proteins
Factories	Cells
Main Office	Cell Nucleus
Branching Out	Cell Division
New Branch Locations	Replicated Cells
Product Blueprints	DNA
Blueprint Photocopies	Replicated DNA
Product Specifications	The Genetic Code
Secretary Work	RNA Transcription
Work Orders	Messenger mRNA
Assembly Lines	Ribosomes rRNA
Trucks & Forklifts	Transfer tRNA
Raw Materials	Amino Acids
Workforce Laborers	Enzymes
Labor Incentives	Vitamins & Co-Enzymes
Specific Task Performed	Form Peptide Bonds
Utilities / Power Plant	Nutrients / Mitochondria
Usable Form of Energy	ATP
The Manufacturing Process	Protein Translation
Waste Materials	H_2O and CO_2
Finished Product	Proteins

Table-1 Demonstrates an analogous comparison between

a factory setting and a manufacturing process and the cellular synthesis of proteins as a means for understanding DNA, RNA, and their functions in living things. In a nutshell, DNA is the cellular blueprint for making proteins.

Dr. Stephen Langer's unique "Glutathione Precursor Complex" and his "Certified Organic Un-denatured Bioactive Whey Protein" provide us with pure ready-to-use protein in a powdered form. They are hormone-free and processed with low heat to keep their delicate protein structure and individual amino acids from being changed by excess processing, in order to maximize our body's glutathione production.

Two major antioxidant enzymes that protect our cells from free radical damage are Glutathione Peroxidase and Superoxide Dismutase. Cells containing the lowest levels of these antioxidant enzymes had more telomere shortening and the highest amount of protein carbonyls.

Telomeres are lengths of protein-coated DNA located at the ends of the chromosomes to protect them from damage such as unraveling or fusing to each other. This short stretch of DNA, like the plastic-coated ends of shoelaces, is not essential to cellular functioning but it serves in self-defense of the chromosome structure and the DNA molecule. Telomeres also provide jumping-on and jumping-off places for the enzymes, which control DNA self-replication and transcription of DNA into RNA.

The concentration of antioxidant enzymes in the cell determines the length of the telomeres in each cell. Researchers have discovered that assessing telomeres is an excellent method for determining the amount of antioxidant enzymes in our cells.

The main cause of telomere shortening is a decreased concentration in the antioxidant enzymes glutathione peroxidase and superoxide dismutase. Deficiencies in these antioxidants and subsequent shortening of telomeres serve to induce and enhance the aging process, along with exacerbating the diseases and illnesses associated with aging.

As our cells divide and the strands of DNA split up (unzip) and replicate to form two new cells with a full complement of DNA, some of the DNA near the ends of the molecule is destroyed. This effectively shortens the telomeres with each subsequent DNA replication and cell division.

This is a side effect of normal cell division but it is not essential to the cell's normal functioning. Telomere destruction is not critically important to normal cellular activity. However, it is critical to the aging process.

Telomeres have a shortening mechanism that normally

limits cells to a fixed number of cell divisions. Research indicates that this is responsible for aging on the cellular level and which effectively sets a limit on life span.

Cell lines frequently end after a set number of cell divisions when their successively shortened telomeres are no longer available to attach the necessary telomerase enzymes; and cells are no longer able to reproduce as necessary for growth, repair, and longer life.

Each time cells divide, their telomeres are shortened. This process continues until the telomeres cannot be shortened anymore. This is regarded as the senescence phase whereby the cells stop dividing and renewing themselves. It is the cause of aging as well as eventual cell death throughout the body.

Telomeres rather directly set the age limit of our life spans. Therefore, if we can feed telomerase enzymes to our telomeres, we can prolong the life of our telomeres and thereby reverse or hold off some of the aging process and increase our life spans.

It is most fortunate that our God-given bodies contain telomeres on the genes of our chromosomes in our cells. If the telomeres were not present at the time our cells divided, we would lose critical genetic material and quickly come to the end of our existence. As long as telomeres are present, our cells will continue to divide and will not lose any of their genetic information.

Since our telomeres become smaller every time the cell divides, they could continue to be reduced in size up to a point where they cannot protect the chromosomes any longer. This results in the cells not dividing at all and going into a senescence phase whereby cellular function slows down to almost zero.

As soon as all of our cells go into this senescence phase, the rest of the body follows; and this results in the aging process. Therefore, it is entirely possible to slow down the aging process by slowing down the telomere shrinking process.

Researchers have measured the amount of protein carbonyls in cells, which form from free radical damage to the cells. This means that more protein carbonyls are contained in cells when they suffer from free-radical damage. If we can control free radicals, we can control the shrinking of telomeres and thereby control how quickly we age.

As we mentioned previously, free radicals are particularly unstable and are thereby extremely reactive because they are missing an electron. Therefore, they move around searching for another electron and they steal it from somewhere else to rebalance themselves.

The electrons can be stolen from any cell they meet, whether it is the heart cells, kidney cells, liver cells, and you name it. When a free radical attacks one of our healthy cells, that healthy cell often dies and accelerates our aging process, which can result in serious illness and eventually lead to death.

Of all the 24,500 genes in our DNA, resveratrol switches on the gene, which regulates aging. In 1993, the discovery of the age-related gene was made by Dr. David Sinclair of Harvard Medical School and Dr. Leonard Guarante of MIT, and was named Sir 2.

Nearly identical copies of this gene are known to exist in all humans and animals. When this Sir 2 gene is activated into use by the resveratrol in red wine, it can reset our body's biological clock. (Resveratrol supplements can be bought from your local health food and supplement store.)

Chapter 7
The Cause of Cancer and Every Other Disease

The health sciences have been searching to find the primary physical causes of all diseases and basic cures for all of them… so-called "magic bullets". After many years, some magic bullets have been found but often are difficult to accept because their simplicity makes it seem that we should have been using them long ago.

Our diet and our environment contains more than 80,000 toxins and chemicals, which are registered with the Centers for Disease Control (CDC).

Our body does a good job of eliminating most of them with its own natural detoxification system, to keep us in good general health. That detox system includes the GI (gastro intestinal) tract, liver, kidneys, bowel, lymphatic system, and others.

This detoxification system slowly becomes desensitized and ultimately compromised by our environmental chemicals and poisons. This can cause us to suffer with chronic fatigue, headaches, food cravings, weight gain, stuffy head, reduced mental clarity, low sex drive, trouble sleeping, and weight gain, which all can result in disease.

Some people are beginning to realize that our modern agricultural practices and food processing methods are the cause of most disease in our world. Some groups of health-conscious individuals are trying to have government mandate and set limits on white flour, wheat, sodas and candy. However, this is not likely to happen soon, because there is big money to be made in selling us mass quantities of food devoid of any real nutritional value or health-improving benefits.

The greatest cause of death in America can be attributed to prescribed drugs and inadequate medical care. The second greatest cause of death in America is heart and blood vessel disease. Osteoporosis, or arthritis and joint disease cause our greatest pain and disability.

In my second book, ***Live Forever: Or At Least to 100***

(Tasseff, 2010), we introduced the concept that cancers and all other degenerative diseases are caused from oxygen starvation within our body.

Oxygen is the most critical element required for Human life and is the key to good health. A strong correlation between insufficient oxygen and disease has been firmly established.

Dr. Otto Warburg was awarded the Nobel Prize in 1931 and again in 1944 for discovering the cause of cancer. He said, "Cancer has only one prime cause. The prime cause of cancer is the replacement of normal oxygen respiration of body cells by an anaerobic (oxygen-less) cell respiration."

Our cells function by burning sugar (glucose) in oxygen to provide energy and results in the waste products carbon dioxide and water. If insufficient oxygen is present at the cellular level, the burn will be incomplete, thereby causing the anaerobic fermentation of sugar to produce carbon dioxide (CO_2) and lactic acid as byproducts of inefficient combustion metabolism.

Since 1926 and due to the work of Dr. Otto Warburg, it has been known that as soon as the available oxygen to a cell drops to below 60 percent of the cell's optimal oxygen requirement, its mitochondria are compromised and hence, its respiration is irreversibly damaged. The oxygen deficient cell tends to become anaerobic and all aspects of normal functioning are afflicted.

Under anaerobic conditions, cells are switched forcibly from oxidation for energy production to fermentation, which is an inferior and inefficient method of energy production. Under these adverse conditions, cells become damaged and they may begin to reproduce copies of themselves wildly and out of control. This is known as cancer.

Dr. Warburg made it known that if any substance deprives a cell of oxygen it is a carcinogen, if the affected cell is not killed. In 1966, Dr. Warburg mentioned that it was useless to search for new carcinogens due to the fact that each carcinogen is the same as the next in that they ALL produce the same adverse results: cellular oxygen deprivation.

The search for new carcinogens has obscured the prime cause of cancer, which is the lack of cellular oxygen.

Dr. Manfred Von Ardenne was born in Hamburg, Germany on January 20, 1907 and was a student of Dr. Otto Warburg (three time nominee for the Nobel Prize and the winner of two). Dr. Manfred Von Ardenne was a physicist who was also a Nobel Prize laureate. He won the coveted Stalin Prize, the Soviet equivalent of the Nobel Prize. In his book, *Oxygen Multistep Therapy*, Dr. Von Ardenne demonstrated that it is possible to bring our oxygen capacity back to what it was when we were young.

The following information is based on Dr. Von Ardenne's research.

If we compare the body of a 25-year old to the body of a 75-year old, we will see that the 25-year old body is better at utilizing oxygen than that of the 75-year old.

Many doctors believe the aging process causes our body to use oxygen less efficiently. However, the exact opposite is true because when our body uses oxygen less efficiently, that is precisely what causes aging and the many health problems that accompany old age.

Since oxygen is the most important fuel of life, it is the nutrient required for every biochemical process occurring in all of the cells in our body. Therefore, it is quite apparent that as the body becomes more efficient in its use of oxygen, it becomes stronger, more energetic, and is capable of reversing the aging process.

To understand how this process takes place, we must know how oxygen gets from our lungs to every cell in our body. I will try to simplify this explanation as much as possible.

One ATM (atmosphere), the measure of our atmospheric pressure, is equal to 760 Torr with about 20% of that pressure due to oxygen. Torr is a unit of pressure named after E. Torricelli, inventor of the mercury barometer, and is equal to a one-millimeter rise of mercury in a glass tube.

This means the oxygen's partial pressure represents 20 percent of the 760 Torr pressure and thereby represents 150 Torr of pressure. This means that the air entering our lungs contains that 20 percent of oxygen at partial pressure of 150 Torr.

As a result, Oxygen in our lungs becomes considerably diluted with the carbon dioxide that is leaving the body as they are exchanged in our lungs during the exhalation portion of our breathing process. This necessitates that the partial pressure of carbon dioxide be subtracted from the 150 Torr of oxygen pressure inhaled.

This leaves us with a remaining balance of about 95 Torr pressure of oxygen in the air sacs (alveoli) of our lungs to push the oxygen into the blood thereby causing the blood to take oxygen through the arteries, vessels, micro vessels, and veins to feed the capillaries, which in turn feed every cell in our body.

During our youthful and ideal conditions, as a 30-year old for example, pressure of the oxygen in our arteries

THE OXYGEN LEGACY

will closely match the pressure in the air of our lungs. While in our youth, the arterial pressure runs about 95 Torr.

As we continue to age and advance into our 70s, our arteries will have only about 70 Torr of oxygen pressure. This is important because the blood carries oxygen to the capillaries but the oxygen must first be dissolved in our body fluids, in order to reach our oxygen thirsty cells that are to be fed by our capillaries. Since oxygen is more difficult to dissolve in liquids than carbon dioxide, the solubility of oxygen depends greatly on the pressure driving it. This is a significant factor.

As venous (deoxygenated) blood exits our capillaries, a difference between the oxygen pressure in the venous and arterial blood that reaches the cells is exhibited. This difference in pressure shows how well the oxygen is being delivered and consumed. Therefore, at 30 years of age, the amount of oxygen released to our cells is much higher than when we reach 70 years of age.

EXAMPLE: A 30-year old will release 55 Torr pressure (95-40=55Torr) and a 70-year old will release only 35 Torr of pressure (70-35=35 Torr). This represents a drop from 55 Torr to 35 Torr. A drop from 55 Torr to 35 Torr represents a drop of 36% in the oxygen pressure that cells are receiving.

When a conventional doctor measures the amount of oxygen in our blood and the test results come back normal, the doctor is missing how well that oxygen is transferred to the cells.

As we age and our oxygen pressure falls, our oxygen level may remain the same in our blood, but there is not enough pressure to push that volume of oxygen to be of optimal benefit to our cells.

In other words, we may have plenty of oxygen saturation in our blood but that does not mean that there is enough oxygen getting into our cells. This is very likely due to the body's inability to transfer oxygen to our cells, which then become increasingly damaged as we age. Therefore, the older we get, the more damaged our oxygen transfer system becomes and thereby makes us more likely to become ill as we age.

There are also many factors, which restrict the optimum amount of oxygen from getting into the blood to be delivered to the body's cells, one of which is hardening of the arteries. The 18 % arterial blockage due to cholesterol buildup in the average person restricts the flow of blood.

There are also many toxins and pollutants contaminating the body's cells and which block the pathways to the cells and thereby further limit the amount of oxygen being delivered.

Armed with this knowledge, it is wise for us to obtain as much oxygen as possible to maintain an optimum level of 60% useful oxygen to bathe all of our cells and in order to prevent cells from becoming atypical and causing disease.

Following, are a variety of comments from various researchers and medical professionals supporting the hypothesis that the gradual decreases in oxygen in our atmosphere and reaching our cells can lead to a great deal of harm including most diseases and cancer in particular.

Dr. Wendell Hendricks of the Hendricks Research Foundation writes, "Cancer is a condition within the body where the oxidation has become so depleted that the body cells have degenerated beyond physiological control. The body is so overloaded with toxins that it sets up a tumor mass to harbor these poisons and remove them from general activity within the body."

Hendricks further states, "The true cause of allergy is a lowered oxidation process within the body, causing the affected individual to be sensitive to foreign substances entering the body. Only when the oxidation mechanism is restored to its high state of efficiency can the sensitivity be eliminated."

Dr. Albert Wahl states, "Simply put, disease is due to deficiency in the oxidative process of the body, leading to an accumulation of toxins. These toxins would ordinarily be burned in normal metabolic functions."

Dr. Spencer Way, in the *Journal of the American Association of Physicians* contends, "Insufficient oxygen means insufficient biological energy can result in anything from mild fatigue to life-threatening disease. The link between insufficient oxygen and disease has now been firmly established."

Dr. Parris Kidd, Ph.D. author states "We can look at oxygen deficiency as the single greatest cause of all disease." He states further, "Oxygen plays a pivotal role in the proper functioning of the immune system; i.e. resistance to disease, bacteria, and viruses."

Dr. Stephen Levine, renowned molecular biologist, geneticist, and author reports in *Oxygen Deficiency, A Concomitant to all Degenerative Illness*, that, "In all serious states, we find a concomitant low oxygen state… Low oxygen in the body tissues is a sure indicator for disease… Hypoxia, or lack of oxygen in the tissues, is the fundamental cause for all degenerative disease. Oxygen is the source of life to all cells. We can look at oxygen deficiency as the single greatest cause of disease. Thus, the development of a shortage of oxygen in the blood could very well be the starting point for the loss of the immune system and the beginning of feared health problems such as cancer, leukemia, AIDS, *candida*, seizures, and nerve deterioration."

Dr. John Muntz, Nutritional Scientist states, "Starved of oxygen the body will become ill, and if this persists it will die. I doubt if there is any argument about that."

Dr. Paavo Airola contends, "An insufficient supply of oxygen to the tissues is linked with such serious conditions as heart disease, anemia, acute poisonings, etc. Many scientists believe that a periodic lack of oxygen must be held responsible for the formation of cancer cells, thus being one of the causes of cancer." He also states, "Each cell of your body is a complete living entity with its own metabolism -- it needs a constant supply of oxygen and sufficient nourishment."

Dr. Norman Mc Vea says, "When the body has ample oxygen, it produces enough energy to optimize metabolism and eliminate accumulated toxic wastes in the tissues. Natural immunity is achieved when the immune system is not burdened with heavy toxic buildup. Detoxification occurs when oxygen is introduced into the system."

Dr. Arthur C. Guyton, M.D., author of *The Textbook on Medical Physiology* suggests, "All chronic pain, suffering, and diseases are caused by a lack of oxygen at the cell level."

Dr. Kurt Donsbach, D.C., N.D., is an educator, scientist, lecturer, consultant; author of *Super Health, Oxygen-Oxygen-Oxygen*, and of more than 50 other publications on the subject of health and nutrition. He is Founder and Executive Director of Medicine at Hospital Santa Monica, Rosarita Beach, Baja California, and the largest holistic hospital in the world; also serves as Medical director of Institute Santa Monica, and Kamien Pomorski, Poland, the sister establishment of Santa Monica. Dr. Donsbach states, "One of the most overlooked benefits of extra oxygen in the tissues is their ability to detoxify more efficiently."

In the *Journal of Experimental Medicine*, Dr. Harry Goldblatt states, "Lack of oxygen clearly plays a major role in causing cells to become cancerous."

Dr. Ed McCabe, author of *Oxygen Therapies* says, "The large majority of these infectious microbes that cause us so much illness and pain are ANAEROBIC -- A big word that means they live and proliferate best in environments where there is LITTLE OR NO OXYGEN." He also contends, "Illness is the result of improper removal of toxins from the body. Oxygen is the vital factor, which assists the body in removing toxins." McCabe further suggests, "Our bodies were designed to function with double the amount of oxygen than is available in today's atmosphere. Deep core ice drillings were up to 38 to 50 percent oxygen: yet today's atmosphere is only 20.9 percent oxygen: and even less in the cities."

Dr. Alexis Carrel, a Nobel Prize winner, believed that the cells could live indefinitely, if the cells are fed nutrients along with oxygen and removing the toxins from the cells. If the nutrients can't enter the cells to feed them and the toxins aren't removed, the cells will soon begin to die due to poisons from their own waste products. For the critical work of feeding and cleaning out toxins from the cells, they must be bathed in a clean fresh useable form of water in the body.

It is clear that oxygen at optimum concentrations is not only fundamental to our normal and immediate metabolic activities, but it is critical for detoxifying our bodies, preventing aging, and eliminating diseases of every kind.

In order for our body cells to function efficiently and to survive, they must be able to convert the molecule Pyruvate (pyruvic acid) into Acetyl Coenzyme A (Acetyl Co-A), one of the intermediary compounds produced during the Krebs Cycle chain of reactions of respiration in converting food (glucose) to energy (ATP) in the mitochondria of our cells. If our cells are unsuccessful in doing this, they are compromised in their ability to use oxygen.

Compromised cells are forced from an aerobic (using

oxygen) state into an anaerobic state of fermentation (using no oxygen) and can become atypical i.e cancer.

An anaerobic metabolic environment eventually compromises everything in our body that is essential for life, such as amino acids that are the building blocks of proteins and which are also the building blocks of life by comprising our tissues, bones, muscles, ligaments, tendons, organs, glands, hair, nails, and most body fluids.

Enzymes, hormones like insulin and the oxygen transporter hemoglobin are also proteins, which can only be synthesized properly under healthy normal aerobic conditions. The lack of sufficient oxygen and the ensuing anaerobic environment will lead to a compromised immune system, premature aging, abnormal cellular metabolism and poor or atypical cell development… cancer… and ultimately an early, untimely, and unnecessary death.

Chapter 8
DCA: A "Magic Bullet" Cure for Cancer

In 2006, cardiologist Dr. Michelakis reported that DCA (Sodium Dichloroacetate Acid) is possibly the greatest cancer cure in history, which is very inexpensive and not owned by any money-hungry organization or Big Pharma. DCA is an inexpensive and essentially harmless chemical, which does not exist in nature.

The discovery of this non-toxic chemical with its ability to kill practically any and every type of cancer (without risky or complicated procedures like chemotherapy, radiation, or surgery) may just be the magic bullet that science and medicine have been searching for. DCA's molecular structure is similar to that of the vinegar (acetic acid) that we enjoy on our salads.

Children in Canada have been treated successfully for more than 30 years with DCA for inborn errors of metabolism due to certain mitochondrial diseases. Eventually, DCA caught the attention of Dr. Evangelos Michelakis of the University of Alberta in Edmonton, Canada, as a possible treatment for cancer.

Over 80 years ago, Dr. Otto Warburg, a German biochemist discovered that tumor cells are the effect of metabolic disorder in healthy cells that cause the cell to become atypical due to a lack of the optimum amount of required oxygen. According to Dr. Warburg, tumors should be understood as a disturbance in the cell's mitochondrial function because the tumor cells do not use oxygen to produce energy.

In the absence of sufficient oxygen, the normal aerobic respiration process of normal cells (using oxygen) reverses itself to the anaerobic fermentation process (using no oxygen), in an often-futile attempt to survive. Rather than dying and in a last ditch effort to survive, a cell fighting for its life will prefer to live in a cancerous state if it can.

Otto Warburg made it known that as soon as the available oxygen to a cell becomes less than 60 percent as required by the cell, its respiration is damaged irreversibly. The cell goes haywire and becomes anaerobic. When this occurs, they are forcibly switched from oxidation for energy

THE OXYGEN LEGACY

production to the fermentation process, which is an inferior method of energy production. This cell can never return to its former state of oxygen respiration. Thereafter, this cell reproduces numerous but atypical copies of itself. This is the condition known as cancer.

Dr. Warburg won his first Nobel Prize in 1931 and a second Nobel Prize in 1944. This important discovery from Dr. Warburg's research was soon forgotten by mainstream science and medicine along with the passing of years. During the ensuing decades, scientists believed that the mitochondria of tumor cells are damaged irreversibly.

Dr. Evangelos Michelakis pondered over Otto Warburg's theory for years. In 2006, he asked, "What would happen if the normal functioning of mitrochondria could be restored?"

Since every living thing has a defined lifespan, our body's individual cells also have defined pre-ordained life spans and can live only so long before they are obliged to die and are replaced by new cells.

If there were not some kind of cell growth limit built into our cells, we would grow uncontrollably. Therefore, all of our cells contain a system to determine when it is time to die thereby initiating that destruction phase known as "apoptosis".

DCA had been used successfully in the science and medical field to treat diseases with connections to mitochondria. For almost 80 years, researchers knew that cancer had a negative influence on mitochondria and caused them to function abnormally.

During most of this time, the popular belief was that, it is not possible for mitochondria to function normally after they have been affected by cancer.

When Dr. Michelakis hypothesized that DCA may restore the mitochondria back to their normal state, he hoped that his DCA experiments would cause the mitochondria to produce an enzyme to help in their own restoration. His expectations were surpassed with the results of his experiments. DCA prevented the devastation of the mitochondria and decreased tumor growth in test tubes and in animals, without affecting healthy tissues.

Dr. Michelakis hypothesized that our body had lost control of its ability to kill cancer cells and have them replaced by healthy new cells, until he demonstrated unequivocally that DCA does in fact bring about the reduction of breast cancer, lung cancer, and brain tumors, as well as other forms of cancer.

It is the mitochondria, the energy-producing powerhouses of our cells, which are ultimately responsible for cellular self-destruction (apoptosis) when cells become old or damaged beyond usual control.

The normal process of old cells dying off and being replaced by new cells is normally a part of our cellular life cycle that keeps us healthy. Cancer is very difficult to treat because the cancer has the power to turn off the cell's ability to die a normal death and thereby makes the cancer itself, in a sense, immortal. This process is controlled by the mitochondria.

Cancer cells have found a way to avoid apoptosis whereby they continue to grow uncontrollably, and which is typical of cancer cells. Cancer cells wouldn't be a problem if they went through the usual apoptosis stage like every other healthy cell because they would also have the control of normal growth restraints.

DCA is capable of inducing apoptosis in cancer cells. When a cancer cell is exposed to DCA, it uses oxygen more efficiently and dies by the apoptosis process. This means that DCA reverses the cancer process (which has no growth restrictions) back to being normal cells that keep growth restrictions and which cause it to lose its immortality. That is to say, the caner cell dies.

Pure DCA (Sodium Dichloroacetate Acid) has been used in recent medical trials, which have proven that this compound can reactivate the mitochondria and restore a cell's original and normal functions, including cell-death or apoptosis and which thereby causes the tumor to shrink in size and mass.

DCA causes cancer cells to self-destruct from the inside of the cell and takes away the cancer cell's immortality by restoring its mitochondria. It appears that DCA is selective for curing cancer by attacking the fundamental process in the development of cancer. It is very interesting to see that DCA may be able to treat and cure many forms of cancer without harming normal cells.

After Dr. Mikelakis deliberately infected rats with human cancer, he treated the rats with DCA and found that their tumors were reduced drastically. He found further that DCA kills breast cancer, lung cancer, and brain cancer cells that have been cultured outside of the body.

According to *Newsweek*, "If there were a magic bullet it may be something like DCA." It appears that DCA lives up to its "magic bullet" nickname via its ability to cross the blood-brain barrier and it stands alone in its unique ability to treat brain cancer. (Most brain cancers are composed of malignant gliomas, which include glioblastoma multiform cells and represents about 60% of the most aggressive types of brain cancer.)

The *Journal of Science Translational Medicine* published a study that shows that DCA has the potential to treat glioblastoma, which is one of the most common forms of brain cancer.

Glioblastoma patients without any treatment live only about three months. If patients take the standard treatment, their current survival rate for glioblastoma patients varies from 14 to 16 months.

In Michelakis' initial clinical trial, treatment of five patients with advanced glioblastoma demonstrated that DCA extended the lives of 80 percent of them. They had no further growth of brain cancer after 15 months of treatment, tumor masses shrank, and the cancer cells died. Even though the study was small and there was no placebo control, the results demonstrate a very promising future for DCA in treating brain cancer and other types of cancers.

In Canada, DCA is already approved for the treatment of metabolic disorders due to mitochondrial diseases. Therefore, some doctors still prescribe DCA off label to their cancer patients. Dr. Akbar Khan of Medicor Cancer Centre in Toronto says, "We are seeing about 60 to 70 percent of patients who have failed standard treatments respond favorably to DCA."

In a peer-reviewed paper published in the *Journal of*

Palliative Medicine, Dr. Khan reports, "It's a case report of a patient with a rare form of cancer that had tried other treatments that weren't working, so he came to us for DCA. It was effective, and actually, the results are quite dramatic. He had multiple tumors, including a particularly troubling one in his leg. DCA stabilized the tumor and significantly reduced his pain."

Dr. Khan continued, "We currently have three patients with [so-called] incurable cancers who are in complete remission, and are likely cured, from our using DCA in palliative (non-curable) treatments. We are in the process of publishing these cases."

Under the direction of Dr. Sebastian Bonnet, researchers at the University of Ottawa in Canada performed some incredible experiments using DCA. They used normal lung, artery, and connective tissue cells and compared them to standard laboratory lung cancer cells and brain cells.

They found what they expected; the cancer cells use less oxygen than the normal cells. When they exposed all of the cells to DCA, the normal cells weren't affected because they were already using oxygen efficiently. However, the cancer cells shifted dramatically; and their use of oxygen was completely normal within 48 hours.

This appears to go completely against the prevailing belief

THE OXYGEN LEGACY

that cancer cells have a permanent and irreversibly defective utilization of oxygen.

These researchers also investigated how DCA effects the production of lactic acid. Since cancer cells do not use oxygen efficiently, the result is they produce excessive amounts of lactic acid and that contributes to the spread (metastasis) of cancer.

Since DCA was shown to improve oxygen utilization in the cancer cells so effectively, lactic acid production decreased to the levels of normal cells. This is a significant factor in preventing the ability of cancer to spread. These facts are definitely encouraging. DCA actually brings about cancer cell's apoptosis (cell-death).

As Dr. Bonnet's team exposed various cancer cells to DCA, they discovered that those cells grew only 1/6th as fast as they ordinarily would have. As they counted the number of cells exposed to DCA, there were 600% fewer cells. Therefore, the cancer cells that were exposed to DCA were dividing and growing at a much slower rate, and they were dying at a much faster rate.

Survivin is a molecule that is made by cancer cells and it indicates how aggressive they are and how well they resist the process of apoptosis. If the cancer creates more survivin, it is less likely to undergo apoptosis (normal cell death).

After the research team exposed cancer cells to DCA, the ability of the cancer cells to make survivin had a dramatic decrease to about 10% of what they make normally. These are extraordinary results even though they are all currently *in vitro* tests, which are conducted in test tubes in a lab and not yet in living animals.

Therefore, the next step was taken to determine whether DCA could produce similar effects in living animals. The researchers took a group of lab rats and implanted them with cancer cells. Group-1 received no treatment while Group-2 received DCA two weeks after the cancer had been established and permitted to grow.

They continued to administer DCA in the rats' drinking water for three weeks. After the end of six weeks, cancers in Group-1 were about 10 times larger than that of the DCA treated rats in Group-2. DCA worked right away with no lag-time effects and it stopped tumor growth as soon as DCA was administered. DCA continued to work effectively and measurably until the end of the experiment (three weeks later).

The researchers carried out a second experiment in which they waited a full ten weeks to allow the cancer to take a greater hold on the rats, before they were treated with DCA. Two weeks following DCA treatment, their cancer tumors had stopped growing and were actually getting smaller. The cancer cells were acting more like normal cells. This is of critical importance.

Examining the rate of apoptosis in cancers of the rats treated with DCA, revealed there were practically no cells that could resist apoptosis, which means they were acting like normal cells. Only 1/16th of the cancer cells were still producing survivin, as the researchers had expected.

This is all very good news about an effective treatment for tumors and leading to a cure for cancer. DCA is non-toxic to normal cells; it works immediately; and is very affordable at a weekly cost of about 20 dollars.

DCA is taken orally and is easy for any patient or doctor to use. It also has unbelievably fast and dramatic effects on cancer cells by causing them to change their metabolism from anaerobic back to aerobic metabolism. DCA controls cell growth, mitochondrial metabolism, and cell death through apoptosis in the same way as normal cells.

You almost certainly will not be hearing about DCA and these incredible medical breakthrough studies, described above, on network TV shows or anywhere in the mainstream media because Dr. Bennet's research was published and made known way back in 2007; and at the time of this writing, remain unknown in the mainstream media.

Dr. Dario Altieri, the director of the Cancer Center at the University of Massachusetts Medical School points out that this research indicates control over cancer growth to stop its progress, destroy it, and even make it more vulnerable to other forms of therapy.

If you do happen to hear anything about DCA, despite these and other studies, it will probably be negative, due to Big Pharma and other Big Money powers that must fear the financial effects of an $80 dollars a month treatment for cancer that will compete with their $20,000 dollars per month therapies.

A standard comment from conventional medical practitioners could be expected such as, "It may be somewhat effective, but it is still unproven and should never be used." Treating cancer is highly profitable. Curing cancer is not.

One obvious fact is that DCA is not new to the medical world because it has been given to children with mitochondrial disorders in Canada for the past 30 years to reduce their lactic acid levels.

According to the usual "Big Medicine", "Big Pharmaceutical", and "Big Money" machine's *status quo* and *modus operandi*, DCA has two major league strikes against it:

    1. It is very affordable and

2. It is easily attainable.

Since a little is known about how it works clinically in children, there should be no complaints against using DCA to treat patients with cancer. The FDA allows patients to import DCA for their own personal use but they need to be under the guidance of a physician who knows how to use DCA.

If you are contemplating starting a DCA treatment for cancer, you might consider the following:

In 2008, it was discovered that DCA works more effectively when combining it with caffeinated tea and vitamin B-1.

A patient with Non-Hodgkin's Lymphoma was taking 35 mg/kg (35 mg per 2.2 lb. of bodyweight) with black tea and vitamin B-1. It caused an extremely rapid dying-off (shrinkage) of his tumor but caused some illness as side effect. He lowered his dose to 10-12 mg/kg of bodyweight and the tumor continued to recede at a tolerable rate without further side effects.

Research indicates that patients must not receive too high of a DCA dosage for too long a period. Adult individuals may have problems using dosages at 25mg/kg of bodyweight and above for long periods. People have been known to show side effects even at 14 to 15 mg/kg of bodyweight per day after three to six weeks.

The Dr. Michelakis paper states the DCA is dose-dependent which means, as the dosage of DCA is higher, the response is better. His patent also gives a dose range of 10mg/kg up to 100mg/kg of bodyweight for tumor action. DCA has a half-life in the body of about 24 hours.

If the DCA is effective against most cancers, the dose can probably stay low thereby creating fewer side effect issues. Taking intermittent "holidays" from DCA usage is a good way to lower the DCA levels and to avoid any severe side effects.

There have been numerous reports from people on DCA that they are eliminating their cancers as evidenced by tumor shrinkage; but they also report that they are sleeping much more, and experiencing muscular weakness, especially in the legs.

No mortalities have been reported from taking DCA. Dr. Michelakis patent states that anti-tumor action can be achieved with a dose as low as 10mg/kg of body weight.

It has been recommended that DCA should be taken only once per day. If you prefer, you can split the initial dosage by taking half in the morning and half at night. Research indicates many excellent responses were achieved with this type of once or twice a day treatment.

According to the World Health Organization (WHO): Several cases of mild neuropathy following DCA treatment of 50 to 100mg/kg of bodyweight per day for several months to a year have been reported (Stacpoole et al., 1998 a., 2001; Spruijl et al., 2001). All were completely reversible after cessation of treatment.

In one case, DCA was reinstituted at 25mg/kg of bodyweight per day following the neurological symptoms, and the dose was maintained for 2 years without further evidence of neuropathy (Stacpoole et al., 1998 a).

The following side effects have been reported with doses of 13 to 14 mg/kg bodyweight after 6 to 8 weeks such as:

- Weakness in legs
- Numbness in toes or fingers
- Peripheral Neuropathy: tingling fingers/toes
- Shaking or tremors in hands
- Mild nausea
- More urination
- Ankles swollen

- Anxiety
- Depression
- Breathing heavier than usual
- Sleepiness
- Tingling (neuropathy) in the lips
- Dizziness and balance issues

Side effects should be closely monitored. If you feel numbness or tingling in your fingers, you should stop taking DCA for a few days. Soon after, you can start again at the same or lower dose level. Report any and all side effects to your physician. Any treatment regimen (DCA or otherwise) or any dosage adjustments you attempt should be approved and closely monitored by your oncologist and your other health care professionals.

A Brief History of Medicor Cancer Centres:

In 2007, Medicor Cancer Centres publicly shared their knowledge about DCA treatment of 118 patients for the first time with the rest of the world. They were the first cancer clinic in North America to prescribe DCA "off label" to cancer patients under a fully supervised medical team.

Medicor has consulted with the relevant regulatory bodies

in Canada and are following their guidelines and policies. Medicor Cancer Centres acknowledges that two of their patients brought DCA to their attention and motivated them to begin DCA treatment.

During 2007, DCA was discovered to induce death in cancer cells that had been implanted in rats, while it was not found to be toxic to healthy cells. The research revealed that DCA killed cancer cells by a newly discovered mechanism that appears to be common to several types of cancer.

The DCA does the job of turning on the natural cell suicide system, which is suppressed in cancer cells and which allows them to die on their own. It does this by altering the cells use of glucose, which starves the cancer cell of energy. Newer research further indicates that DCA also kills many other types of cancer cells.

The first formal human cancer research using DCA was published in May 2010 and confirmed that DCA was an effective anti-cancer drug for treating glioblastoma (brain cancer) patients.

As of April 2009, they have treated 347 patients of which most of them exhausted conventional treatment options. By 2012, over 800 cancer patients had been treated with DCA, which is the most of any center in the world.

Due to the emerging clinical trial data, observational data is no longer being collected. However, they are currently focusing their efforts on publishing their findings in reputable peer-review medical journals.

Medicor Cancer Centres informs us that any data they present is not obtained from clinical trials. Their data is based on their observations of patients that they have treated and doesn't meet the rigorous criteria used in clinical research. They are sharing this knowledge to help further patient care and to improve medical understanding and knowledge for DCA as a cancer treatment.

Thus, Medicor has added a "Live DCA Update" to provide real-time updates of their numbers of treated patients and their types of tumors. They always welcome input from any of their patients to help them serve everyone better.

The following information is directly from the Medicor Cancer Centre:

Their treatment regimen generally consists of DCA in a 2-weeks-on and a 1-week-off cycle, which could be modified due to possible side effects (e.g. ranges could vary from 1 week to 3 weeks of DCA followed by a rest period).

Children are sometimes offered continuous treatment.

Typical doses for adults are in the range of 20-25 mg/kg/day for adults and 25-50 mg/kg/day for children. For elderly patients or others with complicating factors they may use 20 mg/kg/day.

The reason they favor cyclic DCA treatment is that it allows them to use higher dosages and minimize side effects at the same time by having a resting-period where DCA can be cleared from the body.

They believe a dose-response relationship exists with DCA (higher doses yield better response), therefore cyclic treatment may provide a higher response rate while preventing the drug from being discontinued due to adverse events.

It also allows them to clearly decide which side effects are from DCA and which are due to other causes (like cancer itself). This can be invaluable for them in helping to determine if DCA should be stopped or may be safely continued.

All of their patients understand that a positive to DCA treatment is not a guarantee and just like most chemotherapies, the individual response varies.

They encourage discussion of treatment options, known side effects, monitoring protocol, and the uncertainty and paucity of knowledge of the long-term effects of DCA in cancer treatment.

They continue to use their criteria for evaluating patient responses after a minimum of 4 weeks from start of treatment. They have chosen the 4-week mark for their analysis to allow time for DCA to work, and to eliminate the placebo effect (which can typically last for 1-2 weeks).

They advise that this is not a standard criterion and other people may choose to use different criterion in their research. The 4-week cut off likely underestimates true DCA response because they have seen patients improve only after 8 weeks of DCA treatment in some cases.

Out of 179 patients checked after 4 weeks, 106 patients (60%) showed a positive response to DCA. They continue to hold the view that DCA is a relatively safe cancer treatment (especially compared to toxic treatment like chemotherapy) and that the use of supplements such as alpha lipoic acid and vitamin B1 (benfotiamine) are helpful in managing the neurological side effects. In some patients side effects are apparent quite soon while others seem to do quite well from several months to 2 years of treatment.

Their observational DCA data continues to show consistent rates of response and mild side effects confirming that DCA has the potential to be a useful cancer treatment plan. They are receiving comments from many physicians indicating increased levels of interest in DCA and increased willingness to support patients who wish to use DCA. They are also receiving positive feedback from physicians around the world who have used DCA and noted positive results.

Based on their observational data they believe that:

- DCA can be an effective component of a cancer treatment program.

- DCA is a viable option for patients who have exhausted conventional therapies.

- DCA is effective against many different forms of cancers.

- DCA is relatively safe but has specific side effects and should be used under medical supervision only.

- DCA is more effective in healthier patients than those with advanced stage disease.

- DCA can interact favorably or negatively with chemotherapy in some patients. This is hard to predict unless a chemo sensitivity test like Chemo Fit is performed.

- Duration of treatment depends on the individual patient. Limiting factors may include the loss of effectiveness or side effects.

- DCA maybe more effective and tolerable in children, but like adults, children may experience hallucinating or emotional changes due to DCA that resolve when the drug is stopped.

They have not previously acknowledged the psychological aspects of DCA treatment or quality of life enhancements. Subjective responses are always hard to report and categorize therefore they have based all of their evaluations on objective and measurable criteria.

Their published reviews on the aspects of DCA treatment indicate that there are a very small number of patients who are unhappy about trying DCA, mainly because they experience significant side effects (such as neuropathy with burning pain).

However, a majority of patients and their families are highly satisfied and uplifted by DCA treatment. The main reason for this is likely the fact that DCA substantially changes the outlook of patients who are deemed end stage palliative care.

Since DCA is a gentle cancer treatment with scientific

merit, patients' hope for survival or life extension is restored without fear or severe side effects (such as vomiting, diarrhea, hair loss, immune suppression, infection or other loss of quality of life that accompanies treatments like chemotherapy).

Even compared with the approved targeted non-chemo treatments, DCA has fewer side effects, and do not appear to result in severe side effects like internal hemorrhage. This subjective aspect of DCA treatment is invaluable and cannot be ignored.

Chapter 9
Lyme Disease: Difficult to Detect and Treat

Since Lyme Disease doesn't always show its typical symptom of a bull's eye rash someplace on the infected person's body, the symptoms of Lyme Disease closely mimic the same symptoms of Parkinson's disease or ALS (amytropic lateral sclerosis), which is also known as Lou Gehrig's disease. It can also mimic more than 350 other medical conditions, including many or all of the degenerative conditions that we may possibly have.

Although most people believe that Lyme Disease is caused by deer ticks, it is also known to be caused by other ticks, fleas, mites, mosquito and bot-flies. It could also be spread unknowingly through human body contact by a person who was already infected with Lyme Disease.

The microbe, *Borrelia burgdorferi*, causes Lyme Disease and is hard to detect. This microbe is a spirochete bacterium, which has long heavily coiled cells that look like spirals and can aggressively lodge themselves in the tissues of muscles, heart, and brain. They can easily penetrate into the brain in as little as three weeks after one is infected with Lyme Disease.

Live bacterial spirochetes of Lyme Disease have been found in urine, tears, blood, semen, vaginal secretions, and breast milk. It has also been found in dairy cattle of the people who are infected with Lyme Disease.

Some researchers believe about 90% of the people infected with Lyme Disease never had the typical bull's eye rash as a symptom. Other symptoms of Lyme Disease include weakness, lack of energy, and a fever, which could be misidentified as a mild case of the flu.

Since the flu is caused by a virus, antibiotics aren't helpful against a virus. Therefore, antibiotics are not prescribed, which might get the bacterial infection of Lyme Disease under control. As the infection progresses it becomes more difficult to get rid of it.

Lyme Disease has been described elsewhere as having three stages, which each have their own symptoms months or years after the initial infection and frequently lead to its misdiagnosis and mistreatment.

The first stage is the infection from the bug bite or human-to-human contact and develops symptoms within three weeks. If the typical bull's eye rash appears, you may be lucky and be among those that are properly diagnosed and treated correctly.

The other symptoms of this first stage are more common than the typical bull's eye rash and are easily mistaken for flu or signs of aging such as fatigue, muscle pain, headache, fever, joint pain in the knees, fever or problems of the lymph nodes.

The second stage of Lyme Disease can show symptoms weeks or months after the infection. Since those symptoms don't appear to have a direct cause, they are usually misdiagnosed and mistreated. The muscle pain becomes debilitating and can last until you are cured of Lyme Disease.

The third stage of Lyme Disease has the most severe symptom of erosive arthritis of your knees and other large joints. Even if you believe you are cured of Lyme Disease, its symptoms can reappear years later and still affect you.

The symptoms may be muscle weakness, occasional upset stomach, back pain, stiff neck, heart problems, sweating at night and insomnia, which can all mimic Parkinson's Disease and ALS (Lou Gehrig's Disease).

Since these symptoms appear a long time after being infected with Lyme Disease and often seem unrelated, it is quite possible that the person will remain undiagnosed, improperly treated, and very ill, all due to the very tough bacteria, which cause Lyme Disease.

Research indicates that the Lyme Disease microbe (*Borrelia burgdorferi*) is different from most other bacteria by hiding in plain sight, evading antibiotics, and biding its time. It is a spiral shaped bacteria and has a very unusual life cycle.

This microbe hides inside of other cells and goes dormant whereby it is protected from the standard two or three week anti-biotic treatment. This treatment kills off some of the active bacteria but is unable to kill the dormant ones, which can hide up to eight months in their new cyst like formations.

Eventually, these cysts leave their hiding places, when the body undergoes stress, and they enter our blood stream in their spirochete form and continue their damaging ways but they also then become more vulnerable to attack by antibiotic treatment.

Some of the powerful antibiotics used for Lyme Disease can cause excessive harm to the body. The Lyme Disease microbe could be eliminated with time and patience by using the remarkable herb known as Cat's Claw, which comes from a weedy shaped vine with claw shaped thorns, in the rainforests of Peru.

Native Amazonian People were known to use the bark and root for centuries to treat ulcers, arthritis, sexually transmitted diseases, and cancer.

The Cat's Claw herb contains anti-bacterial, anti-inflammatory, and immune modulating properties, which increase our body's germ killing power through granulocites (white blood cells). They contain minute granules that hold very powerful enzymes, which destroy many foreign invaders of our body.

Cat's Claw can be obtained in capsule form from health and nutrition stores as well as from herbal, nutritional, and alternative medicine websites on the Internet.

Chapter 10
Memory Loss and Mental Decline

The causes of frequent memory loss and some other forms of mental decline were discovered by researchers at John's Hopkins, Harvard, Duke, Stanford, and UCLA. It appears that it may be possible to reverse years of brain aging and enjoy clear thinking and focus within 30 days.

Scientists know that memory losses are attributed to faulty "brain wiring" that begins in middle age and makes it harder for the brain to send messages from one part to another and which causes memory lapses and cognitive decline. These messages appear to get lost somewhere, which results in suddenly forgetting things that we were doing, such as looking for our car keys or even where we parked our car.

Brain wiring can become dysfunctional due to the nerve cell's protective myelin sheath wearing away as we get older. Nerve fibers begin to fray as our myelin sheath deteriorates, which results in messages unable to travel along our nerves without being scrambled or diverted along their way. As we get older, we become increasingly more forgetful.

Another reason our memories begin to fail is that we also produce fewer neurotransmitters, which are the brain's fuel and chemical messengers needed to enhance learning, promote memory, and calm your mind allowing us to concentrate effectively.

As the myelin sheaths in our brain and nervous system wear out, fewer neurotransmitters are produced. These vital brain chemicals are only produced when a brain cell receives a message. When our brain cells have worn-out, deficient, or missing myelin sheaths, they aren't receiving messages; therefore, sufficient neurotransmitters are not being made.

By the time we reach middle age, we have worn-out myelin and a deficiency of neurotransmitters. In order to stay mentally alert as we age, it is essential that we maintain healthy myelin sheaths to protect and insulate our neurons and that we produce more neurotransmitters to carry impulses between our nervous system cells.

Our whole body and brain are constantly under constant attack from free radicals. Memory lapses, trouble focusing, fuzzy thinking, brain fog, and other changes are happening to our brain, which are all due to decades of exposure to free radicals and toxins.

Free radicals are unstable molecules of pathogenic or toxic origins that do not belong in our body. These free radicals damage our body and brain cells by attacking the mitochondria of our cells, which are the powerhouses and main energy sources of our cells and our body's normal healthy functioning.

This causes a build-up of harmful amyloidal plaques (similar to cholesterol) to form in our brain. Therefore, our brain doesn't convert enough energy to work efficiently and our brain begins to slow down as a result of our brain wiring not working as well as it did prior to middle age.

Naturally healthy people can prevent the natural brain aging process caused by our exposure to pathogens and toxins such as pesticides, arsenic, aluminum, lead, mercury, and others of which happens over a period of decades. There are things that we can do to decrease the deleterious effects of a lifetime of exposure to these toxins both during our younger lives and even later in life.

Supplements for a Better Memory:

During our middle age years, when our brains begin to synthesize fewer neurotransmitters and lower neurotransmitter concentrations such as acetylcholine, which helps us to recall things like people's names, where we parked the car, or where left our keys.

Acetylcholine is needed by our brain, and is provided by the nutrient choline, which gradually decreases as we get older. If we can increase the supply of choline entering our brain, memory can be increased greatly. Choline is very powerful and raises the body's production of acetylcholine thereby creating increased long-term effects in learning ability and in better memory.

More than 20 studies of over 5,000 patients have shown that choline can increase alertness, increase learning, improve mental clarity, and improve memory, even in people affected with severe mental declines. This research indicates that the use of choline can produce a superior brain with more numerous and more functional neuronal connections.

Alpha-GPC or Alpha-Glyceryl-phosphoryl-choline appears to be the more easily absorbed form of choline. Can you imagine what it might do for you, as a reasonably healthy person, after demonstrating such positive effects in people who were affected with severe mental declines?

Recent breakthroughs in research that can make your brain perform, as it did before middle age by using cutting-edge nutrients, such as Acetyl-L-Carnitine, which actually rebuilds worn-out myelin sheaths and increases our production of neurotransmitters.

Presently, there are quite a few of these beneficial nutrients on the market today as a great variety of nutritional supplements and which make it difficult for us to make wise decisions due to their abundant availability.

Acetyl-L-Carnitine (ALC) is an amino acid-like substance that energizes and supports our brain by crossing the blood-brain barrier to get into our brain cells, to repair damaged mitochondria, and which helps our brain to work more efficiently. This can help us to remember names more efficiently, help us to reverse mental decline, and help our brain to work as it did for years before we reached middle age.

L-Carnitine is similar but not the same as ALC because L-Carnitine supports and energizes the heart. Acetyl-L-Carnitine crosses the blood brain barrier and enters our brain cells thereby helping them work more efficiently by repairing damaged mitochondria.

GABA or Gamma Amino butyric Acid is another essential and important neurotransmitter, which plays an important role in stressful situations by helping to balance our emotions, thereby calming our mind and filtering out distractions. It optimizes brainpower by enhancing mental focus and short-term memory.

GABA also repairs nerve cell connections thereby helping our brain to send and receive information within and between its cells much more easily. If our body doesn't make enough of it, we can have trouble concentrating and our thinking becomes not so clear.

Phosphotidylserine (PS) helps speed up our brain for focus and better learning. It is important to keep our brain cell membranes healthy so they can do their job of cleaning out the waste products such as free radicals and toxins out of your brain cells. As this happens, the neurons of your brain can work properly because they are protected more efficiently by their cell membranes. This helps to enhance proper cell-to-cell communication and allows neurons to communicate more easily. If our neurons are not protected and do not work properly, it slows down our brain responses and renders us less attentive and more forgetful.

Phosphotidylserine is a healthy brain fat that is needed in all of the brain's cell membranes. If you begin to notice memory problems, it is important to supplement yourself with PS because it is not found in most foods and your body makes less of it as you get older. One study revealed that nearly 9-in-10 people with memory problems who took PS noticed a large improvement in only 6 weeks.

Vinopectine helps people to recall new information more easily and stay focused by increasing the blood flow into our brain, thereby supplying more needed oxygen to our brain. Each one of our body's cells needs an optimum amount of oxygen to function properly. If our brain cells receive less than their optimum oxygen requirement, we may suffer memory loss and other serious mental decline.

Vinopectine improves eyesight disorders and improves vision. It also increases crucial levels of ATP (cellular energy) within the brain's neurons and it effectively aids the brain's use of glucose. Remember that glucose from the breakdown of our food is the raw material that our mitochondria use to make ATP…the most usable form of energy for all of the cells in our body.

Vinopectine also increases the brain's consumption of oxygen and thereby resists damage to the neurons caused by low oxygen consumption. It also improves the red blood cell's flexibility in the brain and therefore helps to prevent strokes.

Pregnenoline helps induce a wide variety of biochemical functions that are involved in mental and physical well-being. Pregnenoline has been reported to improve immunity, raise energy levels, increase endurance, reduce stress, improve mood, decrease pain, and increase both male and female libido.

Numerous medical studies have reported that pregnenoline also relieves painful symptoms of osteoarthritis and rheumatoid arthritis, relieves chronic joint pain and muscle aches related to fibromyalgia, lowers total cholesterol and LDL levels, thereby improving cardiovascular status, and maintains the brain cells healthy functioning.

Maca Root (Passion Plant) is a powerful herb that effectively normalizes natural hormones in our body, thereby raising both male and female libido. It has a long history of being safe in humans and animals. It is increasing in popularity for men and women over the age of 40 who suffer from male and female menopause-related loss of libido.

Dr. Gary Gordon, former president of the American College for Advancement in Medicine, reports that, "By using the Peruvian root myself, I personally experienced a significant improvement in erectile tissue response." He also reports that Maca Root works by normalizing steroid hormones, such as testosterone, progesterone, and estrogen, that work together in the human body to influence sexual libido. It appears to restore youthful hormonal levels in both males and females.

Experts have reported that when Maca Root is used as directed, it has no adrenal-inhibiting side effects, which are common with the use of most synthetic hormone prescriptions.

Dimethhylglycine can help you feel 20 years younger with its incredible anti-aging properties, healing and metabolism benefits. Dr. James Balch and Phyllis Balch, C.N.C., have recommended its use for over 48 different health conditions. The amino acid Glycine and its cousin molecule Dimethhylglycine virtually restore bodily functions to their optimum cellular levels and enhance most of the other nutrients taken with them, thereby restoring optimal oxygenation levels to cells, tissues, and organs. It also helps to repair a variety of age-related immune system deficiencies:

- Lowers homocysteine, cholesterol, and triglyceride levels.

- Normalizes glucose metabolism.

- Preserves strong heart function under low oxygen conditions.

- Reduces angina in heart patients.

- Improves overall mental alertness.

- Improves physical performance.

- Increases cellular detoxification.

- Improves liver function and much more.

Personally, I use Pharmaceutical Grade Aji Pur Glycine 500 mg veggie capsules twice daily. Glycine is a natural biosynthetic intermediate amino acid (and just one of the twenty or so building blocks of protein) that also acts as an inhibitory neurotransmitter in the central nervous system and is the same grade of glycine used by healthcare professionals throughout the world.

D-Ribose (a basic sugar that comprises the structural backbones of DNA and RNA) is the new energy booster and it aids recovery from chronic fatigue syndrome by producing and increasing the energy production of the mitochondria in all of the cells of our body. It rapidly raises our body's ATP (adenosine triphosphate) levels, which is essentially the pure cellular energy component used in all of the biochemical reactions that constitute Life.

When we lack sufficient D-Ribose, our entire energy conversion system is compromised. Our ATP production is limited; and without sufficient ATP levels, we lack the fuel that is necessary to restore our energy levels naturally. D-Ribose is an absolute energy source and has been used by professional athletes for many years to improve their stamina and to recover lost energy.

In my own personal health and nutritional supplement regimen, I use 100% Pure Ribose 850 mg veggie capsules twice daily.

Blueberry Extract helps us to avoid premature aging due to decades of exposure to free radicals, toxins and other pathogens. If this exposure isn't stopped, it could cause amyloidal plaques to form on our brain, which disables our neurotransmitters and eventually kills off our nerve cells.

This pervasive deterioration of brain cells and brain functioning can be stopped by using any one (or more) of a variety of antioxidants. The inclusion of antioxidant-rich foods in our diets as well as taking antioxidant supplements will serve to thwart off a number of conditions leading to inefficient energy metabolism and energy conversion as well as the effects of premature aging.

Chapter 11
Alzheimer's and Organic Virgin Cocoanut Oil

In my second book, *Live Forever: Or At Least To 100* (Tasseff, 2010), a chapter was devoted to Alzheimer's Disease: Cause and Cure. In light of recent and seemingly miraculous developments in fighting Alzheimer's Disease, I revisit the topic here and present some of the new and promising research, which is much too valuable to be dismissed.

According to the National Institutes of Health, 4.5 million Americans have Alzheimer's. The early onset of Alzheimer's can strike people who are between 30 and 60 years of age.

If you know anyone with Alzheimer's Disease, then you know just how heart-breaking it can be when this disease destroys mental abilities, dignity, and a person's personality. The body of such a person becomes only the shell of their former self.

Even though still technically alive, such an empty shell of a human life seems like the person you once knew has died and although physically present, you see that the person you once knew or loved no longer exists.

Dr. Mary Newport's husband, Steve, developed the first signs of dementia at age 53 and was rapidly sinking into depression. Dr. Newport took her husband to see a neurologist who gave him a Mini Mental Status Exam (MMSE) whereby he was diagnosed as having a mild case of dementia. Steve also had an MRI of his brain, which was reported as being normal. His mental status remained in decline even after he was placed on several FDA approved medications to help slow the progression of the disease.

Dr. Mary Newport vigorously researched the Internet and uncovered the patent application for a new drug with the primary ingredient being an oil compound composed of MCT (medium chain triglycerides). Each of our body's 70 to 100 trillion cells needs glucose as a principal source of energy in order to survive.

Since our brain cells are responsible for up to 60% of all the energy production that goes on in the body, the brain needs a lot of energy. Normally, the brain burns glucose (a simple sugar) to produce all of this necessary energy. Scientists have discovered that as we gradually age, our body becomes less efficient at using glucose to produce energy. This also applies to the people who have developed Alzheimer's, Parkinson's, Huntington's, and other neurological diseases.

About 4 years later, when Steve was 57 years of age, his mental decline had accelerated whereby he required another MRI scan of his brain. At that time, it was found that his brain had shrunk physically in size, which indicated advanced Alzheimer's disease.

Dr. Mary Newport described her husbands condition, "Many days, often for several days in a row, he was in a fog; he couldn't find a spoon, or remember how to get water out of a refrigerator. Some days were not so bad; he almost seemed like his former self, happy with a unique sense of humor, creative, full of ideas. One day I would ask if a certain call came that I was expecting and he would say, "No." Two days later, he would remember the message from so-and-so from a couple of days earlier and what they had said. Strange to have no short-term memory and yet the information was filed somewhere in the brain."

Dr. Nerwport soon took Steve to the Johnny B. Byrd, Jr. Alzheimer's Institute at the University of South Florida in Tampa to have another MMSE. It was about this time that she learned about MCT (medium chain triglycerides) being used in medications, ketones, their healing effects, and an unusual way to increase ketones in the body. She then understood that this might be a most effective way to help patients with Alzheimer's by increasing the body's natural production of ketones and by being on a diet that is very low in carbohydrates.

Researchers used a testing system, Alzheimer's Assessment Scale with a cognitive subscale (ADAS-COG) and found an impressive improvement in memory performance along with other reactions in the brain as the ketone levels of patients with Alzheimer's increased. Dr. Newport saw the promise of this new potential therapy and quickly started her husband on a daily dose of coconut oil.

Soon after coconut oil is ingested, our intestines rapidly absorb its fatty acids. Fatty acids then go directly to the liver where the liver converts them directly into ketones. Ketones are a readily available source of energy and, as it turns out, ketone therapy is a very good treatment for Alzheimer's.

This is what Dr. Newport said, "The following morning, around 9 A.M., I made oatmeal for breakfast and stirred two tablespoons of coconut oil, plus more for "good luck" into his portion. I had some as well, since I cannot expect him to eat something that I won't eat. Shortly after we arrived at the hospital, they whisked him away for the test. That was about four hours after consuming the coconut oil. When he returned, he was very unhappy about his performance."

Laura, the research coordinator, returned shortly thereafter and began to take his vital signs and blood pressure. Suspecting that we were continuing with the screening process, I asked her if she could share his score with us. She asked, "Didn't he tell you? He scored an 18!" This is a 50% improvement after only one dose of coconut oil.

In 2008, Dr. Newport wrote, "It had been 60 days since he started taking coconut oil. He walks into the kitchen every morning alert and happy, talkative, making jokes. His gait (his ability to walk with coordination) is still a little weird. His tremor is no longer noticeable. He is able to concentrate on things that he wants to do around the house and in the yard and stays on task, whereas before coconut oil he was easily distracted and rarely accomplished anything unless I supervised him directly. About one year after starting coconut oil, Steve's gait was now normal, his reading comprehension improved and now he jogs daily."

Anyone experiencing the first signs of dementia, should

see his doctor and ask him to perform Positron Emission Tomography (PET) scans of the brain, which can reveal a decrease in glucose utilization by measuring the amount of glucose that the cells are currently using for energy production.

As we age, our brain becomes less efficient in using glucose. This is also true with the brains of people who suffer neurological disorders such as Alzheimer's, Parkinson's, Huntington's, Multiple Sclerosis, etc. If it is found that their brains aren't able to use as much glucose for energy as healthy brains, this defect can show up in people about 10 years before their first Alzheimer's symptoms appear.

Since the brain doesn't rely on glucose alone to produce energy, it can be made to produce energy from ketones. Ketones can produce about 125% more energy than when our brain uses glucose. Our aging or diseased brains may lose their ability to burn glucose effectively, but they can still burn ketones as effectively as healthy brains.

People with Alzheimer's now have an excellent method for improving brain function on hand. By combining a low carbohydrate diet while taking "organic virgin coconut oil, they can reduce or even reverse the effects of Alzheimer's.

After ingesting coconut oil, it rapidly goes to the liver to supply your brain with the necessary fuel to burn and thereby restores the brain's normal functioning. It may also be possible to prevent Alzheimer's and many other neurological diseases by employing this same method.

When taking coconut oil, it is best to use extra virgin coconut oil by using only one tablespoon in the morning for the first few days, to allow you to get used to it. As soon as you become used to it, you can then start using two tablespoons in the morning and start adding a second dose of two tablespoons in the afternoon. The goal is for you to get a dose of two tablespoons, twice a day.

Dr. Newport used it for her husband by giving him two measured tablespoons and dissolving it in warm oatmeal every morning. Alternatively, you can simply dissolve it in some hot water, coffee, or tea. It dissolves easily and has a very good taste.

When you begin to take extra virgin coconut oil, you can check your ketone levels with Ketostix indicator strips, which can be bought at your drugstore for about $20 for 100 strips. When you dip one strip in your urine, it should turn purple as your body starts making an optimum amount of ketones. As the color gets darker purple, it means you are getting more ketones.

You should check your urine for ketones first thing in the morning after you awaken. You are not likely to see any change at all, which indicates that your body is making very little ketones. You can then start taking the coconut oil and continue to check your ketones in the morning and afternoon.

If you are not seeing ketones, you are eating too many carbohydrates. This means you will have to decrease your carbohydrate intake until the strips are turning a nice shade of purple. You should expect results within two weeks of taking the full dose. Even though the treatment is completely safe, you should notify your doctor.

Also, if the patient is taking any memory-enhancing drugs typically used for Alzheimer's, do not stop them except under the guidance of your doctor. Talk with your doctor about taking a (MMSE) Mini Mental Status Exam or some other test to monitor the progress of the treatment.

To obtain additional helpful and free information about treating neurological illnesses of all kinds by using coconut oil, visit Dr. Mary Newport's website: www.coconut-ketones.com.

Reducing carbohydrate consumption in our diets and converting our metabolism from a sugar-based to a protein and fatty acid and ketone based nutritional strategy is the entire basis of the Dr. Robert Atkins Lifestyle (Atkins Diet) and includes all of the disease-eliminating, memory-enhancing, energy improving, and weight loss benefits such a lifestyle affords.

Chapter 12
Celiac Disease and Gluten Sensitivity

Due to the rising problems associated with Celiac Disease and Gluten Sensitivity, gluten-free foods are increasingly in demand. Even if you don't have Celiac Disease, you may still be gluten sensitive and not even realize it. Celiac Disease and Gluten Sensitivity could be causing your mysterious ailments such as memory problems, migraines, digestive disorders, and skin rashes.

Gluten is a sticky protein found in many cereal grains and it can be a concealed killer if you have trouble digesting it. This condition leads to an over reaction in the immune system. When this happens, gluten sensitivity damages the intestines by causing our own immune system to attack the intestinal villi, which are the tiny capillary-rich fingerlike projections of our small intestine, which absorb nutrients into our bloodstream.

When our intestinal villi are damaged, it becomes more difficult for our body to absorb the nutrients necessary for good health and by allowing undigested particles of gluten protein, toxins, bacteria, and putrefied waste to leak through our gut and into our bloodstream, travel throughout our body, and are responsible for causing various inflammations throughout our body.

This inflammation causes symptoms such as allergies, asthma, anxiety, fatigue, headaches, skin rashes, joint and muscle aches, mood swings, loss of hair, soft teeth, soft bones, malnutrition, and vitamin deficiencies. As the inflammation from gluten continues untreated, it can shorten your life span considerably by up to 4 times faster than normal.

As many as 3 million Americans suffer from gluten intolerance and still many more can't digest gluten and don't even realize it.

People who are sensitive to gluten must eliminate all foods containing gluten for the rest of their lives. This means that we should avoid all foods made with wheat, barley, and rye, which include breads, pastas, cakes, cookies, cereals and gravy to effectively remove gluten and its pervasive autoimmune reactivity.

Gluten can also be found in many other foods such as instant coffee, salad dressings, canned soups, veggie burgers, meat substitutes, cosmetics, vitamins, and medicines. The slightest bit of flour can result in painful reactions such as diarrhea, constipation, leg cramps, headaches, and painful aching joints.

There aren't many doctors who know that you may be gluten sensitive without actually having full-blown Celiac Disease. This concealed sensitivity can be the main cause of many incurable autoimmune diseases.

Therefore, if you're suffering from an undiagnosed incurable autoimmune disease, it may be a good idea to be tested for gluten sensitivity. Gluten Sensitivity and Celiac Disease are not the same illness, which means they could be misdiagnosed and thereby lead to mistreatment of the disease.

Celiac Disease is caused by gliadin, a gluten protein and its ingestion is usually followed by gastrointestinal symptoms including bloating, gas, abdominal pain, diarrhea, and cramping. Celiac Disease is marked by damaged intestinal villi as indicated by biopsy or endoscopic observations.

If you had an intestinal biopsy or endoscope exam that was normal, it would mean that there wasn't any gluten sensitivity at all. Nevertheless, as we have just pointed out, Celiac Disease and Gluten Sensitivity are not the same because gluten sensitivity usually doesn't have any gastrointestinal symptoms. The intestinal biopsies of individuals with gluten sensitivity are mostly normal.

Another difference between Celiac Disease and Gluten Sensitivity is that Gluten Sensitivity is not associated with the intestinal damage and the accompanying increased intestinal permeability.

Researchers have found that certain immune markers (IL-6 and IL-21) were elevated in Celiac Disease but not in patients with Gluten Sensitivity. Another immune marker (TLR 2) was elevated in gluten sensitivity but not in Celiac Disease. Therefore, based on these studies, researchers have concluded that these two gluten-associated disorders… Gluten Sensitivity and Celiac Disease are two different diseases.

It's very important to distinguish between Celiac Disease and Gluten Sensitivity because many physicians just do not realize that it is possible to be gluten sensitive with very few or no gastrointestinal symptoms. Therefore, they frequently and in error, eliminate gluten as a cause of non-gastrointestinal incurable autoimmune disease, which leads to misdiagnosis of a very treatable condition.

Certain incurable autoimmune diseases include disorders such as:

- Chronic Autoimmune Hepatitis
- Scleroderma
- Hashimoto's Thyroiditis
- Ulcerative Colitis
- Type 1 Diabetes
- Grave's Disease
- Addison's Disease
- Pernicious Anemia
- Sjogren's Syndrome
- Virtiligo
- Lupus Erythematosis (Lupus)
- Polymyalgia Rheumatica
- Dermatitis Herpetiformis
- Auto-antibody Hemolytic Anemia
- Celiac Disease

Of all these 15 diseases just mentioned, only Celiac Disease is caused externally by gluten and gliadin in wheat and other cereal grains. The 14 remaining diseases are believed to be incurable autoimmune diseases that are caused internally. It was once speculated and confirmed by later research that gluten could actually cause the other diseases that were thought originally to be from internal causes.

You can determine if you have undiagnosed (or hidden) gluten-gliadin sensitivity by checking your family health history to find if any members had any of the listed immune problems that haven't been diagnosed. In which case, you might have undiagnosed gluten-gliadin sensitivity and should consider having yourself checked with the secretory IgΛ (SIG) anti-gliadin antibody test.

This test appears as positive in over 90 percent of the people with any of these problems. Many individuals soon have a very noticeable improvement in their health when they eliminate gluten and gliadin, as well as milk and other dairy products.

The most convincing proof of having a problem with gluten sensitivity would be the very noticeable health improvements in any of your incurable autoimmune undiagnosed health problems that follow the elimination of foods containing gluten.

More research indicates that there may be a little recognized reason for the apparent spread of gluten sensitivity that can be traced directly back to the use of antibiotics that began in the 1940s.

Our Big Pharmaceutical Companies, along with Mainstream Medicine, are not likely to recognize this at all. Even many naturopathic practitioners are likely to overlook this problem. It appears that groups of medical practitioners acknowledge that the use and excess use of antibiotics are responsible for many *Candida albicans* (yeast) infections.

In 2003, a group of Dutch researchers reported that *Candida albicans* may stimulate the formation of antibodies against tissue transglutaminase and endomysium, other types of antibodies found in many gluten-sensitive individuals.

In 2009, another group of researchers reported a single case of chronic *Candida* infection in a four-year-old boy who also was found to have elevated anti-gliadin antibodies. Treatment with anti-fungal patent medicines resulted in improvement in the *Candida* infection, while at the same time the anti-gliadin antibodies declined. Although not a controlled study, this case study supports the findings of the research reported in 2003.

Improved diagnostic techniques are increasingly finding more individuals with gluten sensitivity. It seems very likely that the use and excess use of antibiotics is leading to many more *Candida* infections and has consequently resulted in many more cases of gluten sensitivity.

Research indicates that your body has thousands of enzymes including one in particular that can break down gluten to help it be digested and thereby avoiding gluten sensitivity. People with gluten sensitivity have much less of this enzyme than other people. This very important enzyme is called DPP-IV (dipetidyl peptidase IV).

This enzyme was first tested by scientists in the lab by mixing gluten from whole-wheat flour with a DPP-IV formula and they found that this enzyme impressively speeds the process of breaking up the molecules of gluten proteins into smaller particles.

This now becomes easier for you, and enables your other natural protein digestive enzymes such as proteases and peptidases to further digest gluten proteins and thereby eliminate their toxicity.

DPP-IV therapy had a significant impact in breaking down and digesting gluten-rich proteins, when taken at the beginning of each meal. It could very well be the next big step for gluten sensitivity instead of the very difficult process of cutting out all gluten in your food. The Gluten Peptide Digesting Enzymes (DPP-IV) can be easily purchased from your vitamin and health supplement supplier.

Chapter 13
Latent Cancer

My recent research indicates that most people have latent cancer, which is well contained by their healthy immune systems, and it never causes a problem unless it becomes a clinical or detectable (malignant) cancer. Latent Cancer demonstrates the effectiveness of an immune system operated at its optimum efficiency and which stops cancer.

Various published autopsy studies suggest that every one of us over 60 years of age has at least two latent cancers living in our bodies, which are undetected and undiagnosed.

At my current 81 years of age, that tells me that I am one of those people that still have at least two undiagnosed latent cancers. Even though they have not been diagnosed or detected by conventional medical tests such as MRI, PET, or CT scans, etc., that does not mean they are not there. They could be in our liver, colon, lung, stomach, pancreas, or elsewhere. Their locations are unknown because they are latent and the immune system is doing a miraculous job of fighting them.

Another study indicates that by the time women reach 40 years of age, they have a 40 percent chance of having a latent undetectable breast cancer. Even though this amounts to nearly 50% of women that have cancer cells in their breasts, it really isn't bad news because they are shown to be very common latent type cancers, not full blown detectable or clinical (malignant) cancer, and under the natural control of their immune systems.

However, what happens when your immune system is not working at its optimum level? You shouldn't be surprised if one of your latent cancers develops into a detectable malignant cancer within a few years whereby it becomes very difficult to treat. The good news is that there are things you can do for yourself and for your loved ones to prevent this from happening.

It is always important to maintain a healthy lifestyle to maintain an optimum immune system. There appears to be very little doubt that we can greatly reduce the possibility of dying from cancer if we maintain our immune system at its optimum level.

When a person visits his or her doctor for a routine checkup he may be advised to have various tests, which may include MRI, CT, and PET scans. These would allow the doctors to see inside the body in minute detail and obtain a lot more information. However, the doctors don't always know how to interpret this new information. Because of this, over-diagnosis and over-treatment take place in many phases of medicine.

Doctors are to blame but they may justify this by their fear of malpractice and they use unnecessary tests, diagnoses, and treatments for conditions that were never serious or life threatening. Doctors who over diagnose and over treat patients are also making a lot of money fraudulently. Cancer... whether real, perceived, made up, or imagined... pays and pays well!

Many patients may believe that they are overly cautious about their health and request all screenings available to them or they give full responsibility for their health to their doctor and thereby undergoing any tests their doctor orders.

The MRI, CT, and PET scans are tests allowable within the profession of conventional medicine. MRI (Magnetic

Resonance Imaging) uses magnetic fields to create three-dimensional images and doesn't involve using any X-rays or ionizing radiation. This isn't so bad but the CT or CAT scan uses X-ray scanning with radiation from hundreds of different angles to obtain three-dimensional image angles.

The PET scan also uses radiation or nuclear medicine imaging to produce three-dimensional, color images of the body.

Since conventional medicine has no test that will definitively find latent cancer in your body, the AMAS (Anti Malignan Antibody in Serum) test is the best test presently available to detect cancer in your body and it does so at least 19 months before cancer can be detected by the MRI, CT, and PET scans.

According to a recent study in the *New England Journal of Medicine*, one of 80 patients that receive CT scans could directly develop cancer because of the testing. This result is attributed to the dangers of massive amounts of radiation caused by Computerized Tomography (CT scans). This means that 14,500 people could die every year because of merely going along with their doctor's orders!

Women and young 20-year-olds receiving CT scans double their risks for developing cancer. Another study from

Harvard University's Brigham and Women's Hospital revealed that 4 percent were exposed to the equivalent of 2,500 X-rays. That is not difficult to do when every single CT scan delivers the amount of radiation equivalent of 50 to 250 X-rays.

Researchers know that some people have received as little as 5 and up to 38 CT scans. Most people will never know if they have cancer due to X-ray radiation because it can take as long as 20 to 50 years to develop.

As discussed at length in my previous two books, the AMAS test is the only test currently patented that can detect cancer at least 19 months earlier than any other test and without the risk of radiation exposure. I strongly recommend the AMAS test every few years as one more preventative strategy in your health defense arsenal.

Chapter 14
The FDA and Its Approved Cancer Drug: Avastin

In Chapter 14 of my second book, ***Live Forever: Or At Least To 100*** (Tasseff, 2010), we introduced the *New York Times* report that oncologists (cancer treating medical specialists) are being paid kickbacks by the pharmaceutical companies in order to prescribe their questionable drugs. An oncology group of six doctors received $2.7 million in kickbacks in only one year for drugs, but their identity was not revealed of course.

The cancer drug Avastin (Bevacizuman) was first introduced in the United States (as its first market) by the pharmaceutical giant, Roche. This was accomplished with the help of the US government, through our tax dollars, by sponsoring the drug's research, which eventually helped it to receive a patent.

Roche's U.S. government-sponsored trial of the drug began in early 2005 in the United Kingdom, Germany, and Switzerland. It is also very interesting to know that, after receiving their patent, Roche and Guenentech (Roche's co-developer of Avastin) were at complete liberty to name their price tag for the drug. Guenentech priced the drug at $4,400 a month at first, which was about $1,000 more than its price in the United Kingdom. Avastin could cost anywhere from $4,400 to $8,800 a month, depending on the treatment.

According to the *New York Times* (February 15, 2006), a year's cancer treatment with Avastin costs $100,000. Some desperate patients have been known to pay for their treatments by mortgaging their homes and even going broke to stay alive.

If American progress is based upon developing new drugs to fight disease, we as taxpayers pay for it in two basic ways. As taxpayers, we support the research through the National Institutes of Health (NIH) and through federal tax deductions on Research and Development (R&D) costs of the Pharmaceutical Industry.

As consumers, we support research and development (along

with pharmaceutical company executive salaries) by paying their high prices made possible by their exclusive patents from their government granted monopolies that reward them for the innovative drugs.

A little over 5 years have passed since the U.S. government trials of Avastin, *The Buffalo News* (2011)... "FDA Pulls Approval of Avastin for Breast Cancer", as follows:

"The government delivered a blow to some desperate patients Friday as it ruled the blockbuster drug Avastin should no longer be used to treat cancer: Studies haven't found that it helps those patients live longer or brings enough other benefit to outweigh its serious side effects."

Doctors are free to prescribe any marketed drug as they see fit. So even though the FDA formally revoked Avastin's approval as a breast cancer treatment, women could still receive it; but their insurers may not pay for it. However, "Medicare will continue to cover Avastin", said Brian Cook, spokesperson for the Centers for Medicare and Medicaid Services.

A year's treatment with Avastin can reach $100,000. Over the objections of its own advisors and to the surprise of cancer groups, FDA gave Avastin conditional approval. It could be sold to women with breast cancer while manufacturer Guententech continued trying to prove that it really works.

Ultimately, the tumor effect was even smaller than first thought. Across repeated studies, Avastin patients didn't live longer or have a higher quality of life. Yet, the drug poses some life threatening risks and side effects including severe high blood pressure, massive bleeding, heart attack or heart failure, and tears in the stomach and intestines. The FDA concluded two public hearings in 2011 and 2012 where FDA advisers urged the agency to revoke the drug's approval.

Guenentech had argued the drug should remain available while it conducted more research to see if certain subsets of breast cancer patients might benefit and some patients and their doctors had argued passionately for the drug.

The following is information that was sent to me in a newsletter, *Natural Health Sherpa* dated November 29, 2011, Subject: A startling confession about your health.

Dr. Allen Roses, a top executive and insider of the pharmaceutical giant Glaxo-Smith-Kline and world wide vice president of genetics, admitted in 2003 that, "The vast majority of drugs… more than 90%… only work in 30 to 50 out of every 100 people."

This means that most prescription drugs just don't work on most people who take them. This is the first time that high-ranking pharmaceutical executives have gone public and admitted that most drugs produced by the pharmaceutical industry are ineffective in most patients.

When there is a big conspiracy or cover-up of foul play costing billions of dollars to patients along with loss of lives, it is one of the most obvious practices of fraud on a grand scale. This is one of the largest cases of fraud that you can possibly imagine and perpetrated by the pharmaceutical profession.

It's not just that they sell worthless products but some of them are also killing instead of healing. This could very well be the reason why the majority of doctors are frustrated after entering the medical profession with a genuine desire to cure people but soon find out that their training for treating patients is only with drugs and with surgery.

Research reveals that the average of one man's End-Of-Life-Healthcare-Costs are $618,616 total. Almost 2/3 ($412,000) of it was for the last 24 months, whether being hospitalized or not (at over $17,000 per month).

About 700,000 people are admitted to Hospice each year. Sixty percent (420,000) of these are cancer patients. If even 25 percent of these people were saved and spared from the death sentence, that would be about 105,000 people spared at $600,000 each for a total of 63 billion dollars.

It is painfully and shamefully obvious that Conventional Medicine and Big Pharmaceuticals are most definitely bankrupting our country with greed, lies, deception, and perhaps in some cases, even murder.

Conclusion:
A Legacy of Oxygen for You

I would be remiss at the conclusion of this book if I did not reiterate my main contention as well as that of the most progressive and aggressive workers, researchers, and clinicians in the fight against cancer and a host of other diseases.

Oxygen is the key to our survival, to the fight against cancer, and to maintaining a healthy functioning immune system. The more oxygen that we get, the healthier we will be and the more ready we will be to fight off any opportunistic seeds of disease that invade us or arise from within our bodies.

Anything that we can do to increase our blood flow and the amount of oxygen reaching our cells should be done. In this book as well as in my previous works, we have provided you with numerous methods and options, including nutrition and taking nutritional supplements, which if vigorously employed, will increase your blood flow and get more vital oxygen into your tissues and cells.

In addition to the nutrients and supplements discussed here for improved oxygenation, I strongly recommend a regimen, which includes the following:

- Follow a program of daily vigorous aerobic exercise.

- Practice frequent daily deep breathing exercises to maximize inhalation, exhalation, and exchange of gasses in your lungs.

- Use Breathe-Right brand nasal-opening strips to help maximize oxygen intake. They work!

- Reduce snoring during sleep. Snoring is a symptom of restricted airflow. There are simple devices and techniques to effect better breathing during sleep that are inexpensive and which do not involve surgery.

- Don't stay cooped up indoors all winter. Cold air contains more oxygen. Get outside and breathe in lots of that fresh clean cold air.

- Get lots of fresh air whenever and wherever you can. Go walking out in the countryside often.

- And above all else... DON'T SMOKE!

Postscript:
Disclaimer, Recommendations, and

My intention in writing this book is to share with you what I have learned and employed in winning the ultimate battle for my own health as based upon a lifetime of good living, from conducting my own in-depth research, and from the experience of overcoming my own health obstacles.

My continuing legacy to you is to provide you with the ammunition that I have found available and have used to improve my own general health and happiness.

It is my hope that as you read this book, you will do so with an open mind and find both the information and the inspiration to continue to do your own research, to seek appropriate and cooperative professional medical health care consultation as necessary, and to make informed decisions that will lead you to a healthier and happier life.

None of the information provided nor any of the opinions expressed in this publication should be construed as personal medical advice or instruction. No action should be taken based solely upon on the contents of this book. Readers are advised to consult their own appropriate health care professionals on any matters relating to their personal medical health, health concerns, symptoms, illness, disease, or treatment strategies. This means… "See Your Doctor."

No information contained herein, as expressed, or as implied, or as might be interpreted by the reader, is intended to diagnose, treat, cure, or prevent any disease. That is why the reader is advised again to seek his or her own personal professional medical consultation. I have done my very best to ensure that the contents of this book are accurate.

The information contained herein is based upon my own personal research and personal experience and while I believe it to be correct and accurate as based entirely upon my own research and experience, it cannot be guaranteed in any way to be correct and accurate. No warrantee or guarantee of any kind is stated, intended, expressed, or implied.

While the information provided and the opinions expressed in this book are believed to be accurate and are based on the best judgment of the author, readers who fail to consult with appropriate health care authorities assume ALL risk for ANY injury and for consequences of any kind.

Neither the author, nor the publisher, nor any person associated with the writing, editing, publication, printing, or distribution of this book is liable for any errors, inaccuracies, or omissions.

The reader assumes ALL responsibility for ANY actions taken and is repeatedly advised to seek appropriate professional medical consultation.

Neither the U.S. Food and Drug Administration (USFDA) nor the American Medical Association (AMA) have approved any of the materials contained, practices described, or information presented in this book.

The author does however recommend that the USFDA, the AMA, medicine, big medicine, big drug and pharmaceutical companies, and big money finally admit to us the benefits of natural and herbal remedies which can quickly and cost effectively save millions of our dollars and both prolong and save millions of our lives each year.

About The Author.

Tom Tasseff was born to Macedonian parents in the "Steel City", Lackawanna, New York on April 10, 1931. He was the eldest son and the third of seven children. His proud Eastern European family traditions and upbringing during both the Great Depression and the Second World War contributed greatly to his success, his patriotism, and his strong American work ethic.

During World War II when Tom was only twelve years old, he supplemented his family income by working as a shoe-shine boy. It was at this time that he bought his first fitness magazine, *Strength & Health*, which featured articles by the magazine's editor Bob Hoffman as well as John Grimek, Steve Stanko, and many other early fitness gurus.

As Tom's collection of *Strength & Health* magazines accumulated, he was encouraged and inspired by the monthly features and learned to develop good health habits to maintain a "sound mind and a healthy body".

After graduating from Lackawanna High School in 1950, he went to work at Bethlehem Steel, earning and saving enough money to attend classes at Canisius College in nearby Buffalo, New York. However, it was then that his nation called him to service during the Korean War. Tom was activated into the U.S. Navy Air Corps in which he was already proudly serving as a reservist.

Once activated in the Navy, Tom was fortunate enough to attend the training school of his choice because of his very high scores on the Navy Achievement Tests. He successfully completed his Aerology-Meteorology training in Lakehurst, New Jersey and served as a U.S. Navy Weatherman for four years during the Korean War.

Tom received an honorable discharge in 1955 from his final base of operations at the U.S. Naval Air Station in Columbus, Ohio. Upon Tom's discharge from the Navy, he went back to work at Bethlehem Steel as a trouble- shooting electrician for diversified electrical controls in the Blast Furnace Department until the steel plant's shutdown in 1983.

Not willing to become another casualty of "The Rust Belt",

Tom focused his attention, his hard-earned assets, and his ingenuity on becoming a builder of homes and a developer of residential subdivisions.

Tom's first subdivision was Tasseff Terrace in Hamburg, New York where he built a home for Russell "Rusty" Jones, the physical conditioning coach of the Buffalo Bills Football team. They remained good friends and neighbors until Rusty moved to Chicago in 2004 to become the physical conditioning coach of the Chicago Bears.

After building Tasseff Terrace Subdivision, Tom built the nearby Ridgefield Estates Subdivision and has most recently completed the scenic Castle Ridge Subdivision all in the lovely and quaint little Town of Hamburg, New York where Tom and his dear wife, Nada, currently reside.

Throughout his life, Tom Tasseff has continued his research on health, fitness, and the prevention of disease. He attributes much of his personal and professional success to his healthy body and his healthy mind.

Tom wrote this book to share with you what he has learned and employed over his lifetime in hopes that you too will be encouraged to take positive action and take responsibility for and control of your life, your health, your happiness, and your destiny.

Bibliography:
References Cited and Sources of Further Information.

These are some of the resources that I have read, consulted, or referred to both directly and indirectly during the writing of this book. I recommend these resources to you the reader for more detailed information on any of the topics that have been so briefly touched upon herein.

This book and these further resources will give you a good fighting start in doing your own research and in taking personal control and responsibility for winning the ultimate battle for your health. Best Wishes, Good Luck, and Good Health to You!

Balch, James and Stengler, Mark. 2004. *Prescription for Natural Cures: A Self-Care Guide for Treating Health*

Problems with Natural Remedies Including Diet and Nutrition, Nutritional Supplements, Bodywork, and More. Hoboken, NJ. 736 p.

Balch, J. (Ed.) (monthly newsletter). Dr. James Balch's *"Live Well Naturally Newsletter"*.
www.LiveWellNaturally.com.

Batmanghelidj, F. 1995. *Your Body's Many Cries for Water: Second Edition.* Vienna, VA: Global Health Solutions; 182 p.

Brooks, T.J. 1963. *Essentials of Medical Parasitology.* New York, NY: McMillan & Company. 1963. 358 p.

The Buffalo News. 2011 (Saturday, November 19, 2011, page A9). FDA Pulls Approval of Avastin for Breast Cancer.

Carter, J.P. *Racketeering in Medicine: The Suppression of Alternatives*, Charlottesville, VA: Hampton Roads Publishing Company, Inc. 1993. 392 p.

Clark, H.R. 1993. *The Cure for All Cancers: Including Over 100 Case Histories of Persons Cured.* San Diego, CA: ProMotion Publishers. 1993.

Clark, H.R. 1995. *The Cure for All Diseases: With Many*

case Histories. San Diego, CA: New Century Press. 1995.

Clark, H.R (Website). Hulda Regehr Clark Information Center: www.DrClark.com

Douglass, W.C. (Ed.). Real Health Breakthroughs (monthly newsletter). Dr. William Campbell Douglass. *The Douglass Report*. www.DouglassReport.com.

Duarte, Alex. 1995. *Dr. Duarte's Health Alternatives: Your Exclusive Health Management System* by Alex Duarte Publisher: Morton Grove, IL.: Mega Systems Inc. 1995; Audio Cassette Set With Book. 16 Audio Cassette Tapes and book 444 p.

Fischer, D.S., Knobf, M.T., Durivage, H.J., & Beaulieu, N.J. *The Cancer Chemotherapy Handbook (6th Edition)*. Philadelphia, PA: Mosby. 2003. 640p.

Jensen, Bernard. 2000. *Dr. Jensen's Guide to Diet and Detoxification: Healthy Secrets from Around the World*. Lincolnwood, IL: Keats Publishing. 128 p.

Langsjoen, P.H., Folkers, K. 1993. Isolated diastolic dysfunction of the myocardium and its response to CoQ10 treatment. In: *Seventh International Symposium on Biomedical and Clinical Aspects of Coenzyme Q*. In:

Folkers, K., Mortensen, S.A., Littarru, G.P., Yamagami, T., and Lenaz, G. (eds) *The Clinical Investigator,* 1993. 71:S140-S144.

Life Extension. (monthly newsletter). www.LEF.org

McDougall, J.A. (Ed.) (monthly newsletter). Dr. John A. McDougall's *"To Your Health"* www.DrMcDougall.com.

Rowen, R.J. (Ed.) (monthly newsletter).
Dr. Robert J. Rowen's *Second Opinion.*
www.SecondOpinionNewsletter.com.

Sinatra, S. (Ed.) (monthly newsletter). Dr. Steven Sinatra's *"Heart, Health & Nutrition".* www.DrSinatra.com.

Thompson, J. (Ed.) (monthly newsletter). Dr. Jenny Thompson. *Health Sciences Institute Newsletter.* www.HSIBaltimore.com

Torrey, E.F. 1983. *Surviving Schizophrenia: A Manual for Families, Consumers, and Providers (4th Edition).* New York, NY: Harper Collins Publishers, Inc. 544 p.

Torrey, E.F. 1984. *The Roots of Treason: Ezra Pound and the Secret of St. Elizabeth's.* 1984. London: Sidgwick & Jackson

USA Today, January 11, 1999 America's Goo And Glue Diet.

Wamback, S.J. 1999. *The Third Day: A Geological and Biological Analysis of The Origin of Life On Earth.* Great Lakes Geological and Environmental Sciences. Steven J. Wamback.

Weinberger, Stanley. 1993. *Parasites: An Epidemic in Disguise.* Healing Within Products. 58 p.

West, B. (Ed.) (monthly newsletter). Dr. Bruce West's *"Health Alert"*. www.HealthAlert.com.

Whitaker, J. (Ed.) (monthly newsletter). *Health & Healing: Tomorrow's Medicine Today.* www.DrWhitaker.com.

Williams, D. (Ed.) (monthly newsletter). Dr. David William's *Alternatives for the Health- Conscious Individual.* www.DrDavidWilliams.com

Books by Tom Tasseff:

Win The Ultimate Battle For Your Health:
The Lifesaving Legacy of Tom Tasseff
(Thomas Tasseff, 2008, Outskirts Press, Inc.)

Live Forever (Or at Least to 100):
More Lifesaving Strategies from Tom Tasseff
(Thomas Tasseff, 2010, Outskirts Press, Inc.)

The Oxygen Legacy:
A Fountain of Youth and an End to All Disease
(Thomas Tasseff, 2012, Outskirts Press, Inc.)

CPSIA information can be obtained at www.ICGtesting.com
Printed in the USA
BVOW081749020812

296925BV00005B/63/P